The Art and Practice
of Western Medicine in the
Early Nineteenth Century

A

DISQUISITION ON THE

ART AND PRACTICE OF MEDICINE,

AND AN

ECLECTIC REVIEW

OF

PHYSIOLOGIC PRINCIPLES

AS ESPOUSED IN

WESTERN EUROPE, BRITAIN, AND THE NEW

UNITED STATES OF AMERICA,

1800-1825

BY PROFESSOR CARL J. PFEIFFER

McFARLAND & Co· INC.
Publishers

The Art and Practice of Western Medicine in the Early Nineteenth Century

CARL J. PFEIFFER

McFarland & Company, Inc., Publishers

Jefferson, North Carolina, and London

LIBRARY OF CONGRESS CATALOGUING-IN-PUBLICATION DATA

Pfeiffer, Carl J.
    The art and practice of Western medicine in the early
nineteenth century / Carl J. Pfeiffer.
        p.   cm.
    Includes bibliographical references and index.

    ISBN 978-0-7864-7611-4
    softcover : acid free paper ∞

    1. Medicine—History—19th century. I. Title.
[DNLM: 1. History of Medicine, 19th Cent. WZ 60 P526a]
R149.P45 2013
610'.94   84-43232

BRITISH LIBRARY CATALOGUING DATA ARE AVAILABLE

On the cover: *The Cow-Pock or the Wonderful Effects of the
New Inoculation*, by artist James Gillray (1756-1815), color
engraving published by H. Humphrey, June 12, 1802, London
(Library of Congress)

Manufactured in the United States of America

McFarland & Company, Inc., Publishers
  Box 611, Jefferson, North Carolina 28640
  www.mcfarlandpub.com

To Carl F.H. Pfeiffer, M.D.,
my father,
and family physician extraordinaire

Table of Contents

Tables and Figures

Preface

As a writer and as a medical scientist, I cannot attempt to extol the historiographic virtues or consequences of my pen in the field of medical history. Still, and in spite of any literary deficiencies in the present small book, I hope that the reader will agree that there is a story to be told about early nineteenth century medicine. In modern medical science (and I use this term loosely in historical perspective, because in a few decades most of our present-day methods will become obsolete), our cardiac assist devices, genetic engineering and other sophisticated advances have required the experiments, mistakes, and sacrifices of our forebears in medicine. Though it is easy to examine with humor the beginning stages of medicine as a science, the fundamental natures of pain, death, heartbreak and frustration of patient, relative, or physician have not changed with time. Only the patterns of disease incidence and age-specific morbidity rates, and in some cases the degree of pain or the age of death, have changed. As the reader will find in the numerous quotations included in this monograph, human nature has also changed very little. There is an everlasting opposition between intellectual genius and curiosity on the one hand, and sometimes stubborn over-acceptance of traditional thought on the other hand. Further, this interplay seems always to be modulated by nonscientific and nonhumanitarian factors of political or economic nature.

The period selected for this book, 1800–1825, was chosen on the basis that though few authors have previously concentrated upon this significant period of Western medicine, it was a most important embryonic period for scientific exploration, debate, and experimentation, and one which formed the basis upon which later nineteenth century medicine explosively developed. It was also the first period in Western medical history when large numbers of medical journals began publication; relatively few existed prior to 1800 compared to 1825, and this important fact encouraged an extensive scientific debate less possible earlier by means limited to books, verbal communication, and scientific demonstration. If there should be any virtue in the present monograph, it is that almost all of the contained information has been obtained directly from the original source material, fortunately without the development of a dust allergy on the part of the writer.

The present work was undertaken over a period of many years, since it has been the continuing responsiblity of the writer to teach medical and veterinary students and to tackle in the modern research laboratory, the pathophysiologic basis of selected digestive tract diseases. As a typical medical school professor with a rather peripatetic lifestyle, the author began this work using the excellent historical collection of the Stanford University Lane Medical Library, continued the work while a student at Harvard University, using the outstanding Countway Library of Medicine, and later while a professor at the University of Pennsylvania School of Medicine, the fine old archives at the Library of the College of Physicians and Surgeons in Philadelphia. Later, while a professor at Memorial University of Newfoundland, Faculty of Medicine, the author received the most gratefully appreciated assistance of two Vice President's Research Grants to facilitate further research and writing of this monograph. The later work was done in Cambridge, England, and in the northeastern United States. Some of the illustrations were obtained by the author from original etchings or engravings in England, and a few from the National Library of Medicine in Bethesda, Maryland. The actual writing was accomplished in Boston, Philadelphia, and upstate Maine, in Cambridge and Hampstead England, in Köln, West Germany, and in St. John's, Newfoundland, Canada.

The most important discoveries, when familiarized to the mind, are contemplated with indifference. Who now wonders at the discovery of America, or the circulation of the blood? There is, however, a period between the conception of a discovery and its mature birth, fraught with more pangs than war or women know; and there is no light, in which the human mind can be viewed, more interesting than during this anxious period.
— *Editor,* The Medical and Physical Journal
(London) 5:505 *(1801)*

Chapter I

The Setting for Early Nineteenth Century Medicine

It has been said, quite correctly, that scientific medicine, and indeed the scientific method itself, began in the nineteenth century. In the mid- and final parts of this century there was in fact an explosive growth of most divisions of science in the Western world. For such an intellectual and technical growth to occur, even as with the magnificent development of arts during the Renaissance, there had to be underlying social conditions to nurture such development. Furthermore, the germination of this flourishing midcentury activitiy and progress must be sought, and can be found at the dawn of the nineteenth century. To be sure, medical and physiologic experiments had been performed and reported prior to 1800, and numerous important scientific discoveries had been made prior to that time, but the seeds of scientific medical inquiry and communication genuinely began to take hold and grow in the early nineteenth century. The practice of medicine was very much an art, rather than a science, at this time, but scientific inquiry was becoming evident, and was reckoned with by numerous writers in the field of medicine. These scientific advances in medicine did not occur in a vacuum, but were closely associated with other technological advances in the society.

Political and Social Background

This was an exciting and, at times, promising era in the western world, with much rapid change occurring between 1800 and 1825 (Table 1). The political and economic conditions, which both caused and were affected by the social climate throughout Europe and the British Isles, were greatly influenced by the upheaval due to the French Revolution and Napoleonic Wars (1789-1804). Such political reactions were felt significantly beyond the defeat of Napoleon in 1815. At the conclusion of the eighteenth century, France, with its population of 25 million, was by far the largest body of western people with a single government. There were only 10 million English plus Scottish residents, a similar number of disunited German-speaking people, two million

1

Table 1
Major Political, Economic
and Other Events, 1800–1825

	Europe and Great Britain		*United States of America*
1800	Great political upheaval due to French Revolution and Napoleonic Wars.	1800	President John Adams, Census shows 5,300,000 population, of which 1,000,000 are Negroes, 90% of who are enslaved. Congress opened first session in new capital of Washington. New states are Vermont, Kentucky and Tennessee.
1801	First steamboat on Thames River.	1801	Jefferson becomes 3rd Federalist President, Lewis and Clark expedition begins. Louisiana purchase, economic expansion and westward migration.
1802	Napoleon Bonaparte made Consul for life.		
1803	Defeat of Austria. England declares war against France. Napoleon makes all English in France prisoners of war.		
1804	France and Britain at naval warfare, Schiller writes Wilhelm Tell. Proclamation of French Empire and coronation of Napoleon.	1805	Napoleonic Wars continue to depress American trade and disrupt American politics.
1805	England declares war against Spain. Battle of Trafalgar and death of Lord Nelson.	1807	Embargo Act of Thomas Jefferson.
1806	End of First German Reich. Napoleon declared England blockaded.	1809	James Madison becomes President.
1807	France and Britain practiced search and seizure of U.S. ships and Great Britain impressed American seamen. Jubilee of George III in England. Napoleon invades Portugal. Abolition of slave trade in England.	1810	Census shows 7,239,881 population in 17 states. New England seething with secessionism.
1808	Continued writing by aged Goethe. Regulation of cotton spinners' wages and riots in cotton district in England.	1811	American "war hawks" gain momentum; lack of faith in diplomacy with Britain. Crises with American indians increases.
1809	Imprisonment of Pius VII. Birth of Charles Darwin.	1812	Congress declares war.
1810	Writings of Keats, Hugo, Poe, Thoreau, Longfellow, Wordsworth, etc. Theory of colors published of Goethe.	1815	Treaty of Ghent; improved relationship between U.S.A. and Great Britain.
		1816	Era of nationalism, population spills over Appalachians, increased economic, agricultural and industrial productivity.
		1817	James Monroe becomes President.

Europe and Great Britain

1811 Economic crises in France.
1812 Napoleon leads ill-fated army into Russia.
1814 Collapse of Napoleon's military capability after invasion of Russia and defeat at Leipzig, allows Britain to be more aggressive toward U.S.A. Allied invasion of France, First Treaty of Paris, Congress of Vienna. Metternick is leading Austrian statesman.
1815 Napoleon defeated at Waterloo, Second Treaty of Paris.
1817 Savings banks established in Britain.
1818 Occupation of France ended. Birth of Karl Marx.
1821 Death of Napoleon.
1824 Succession of Charles X of France.
1825 Law against sacrilege in France. Abolition of salt tax in England.

United States of America

1818 Regular packet sailing scheduled between New York City and Liverpool (33 days). Control of Florida by Spain lost to U.S.A.
1819 Westward expansion, financial depression.
1820 Census shows population of 9,638,453, in 22 states.
1823 Disappearance of Federalist Party. Improved economy.

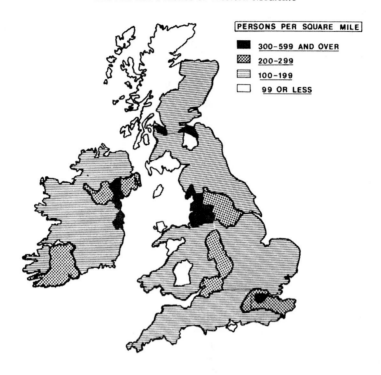

Fig. 1. Population density in the British Isles in 1801. Adapted from a map of G. Melvyn Howe, "Man, Environment and Disease in Britain," 1972, Barnes and Noble, N.Y., p. 153.

Dutch, and three million Belgians in these particular countries.[1]* British subjects, at first inspired by the French Revolution in 1789, rapidly became disillusioned with the violent tactics of the revolutionaries, and by 1803 England had declared war against France, by 1805 against Spain, and by 1812 was at war with the new United States of America. The search for political freedom by many groups in France opposed to despotism had inspired workers in several other Western European countries to consider such a quest. In Germany, though countrymen remained relatively inactive politically in terms of revolutionary fervor, this era was the supreme age of German literature and philosophic thought, the age of Goethe and Schiller, of Kant, Fichte, Hegel, the Schlegels and others. Beethoven, who was a political liberal and champion of the oppressed, had composed his Pastorale and Fifth Symphonies by 1808 and Egmont Overture by 1811. By 1810, the writings of Keats, Hugo, Poe, Thoreau, Longfellow, and Wordsworth had appeared in English. The industrial revolution, which had already begun in England, had started to enhance the concentration of urban residents, especially in the north of

*See Chapter References, beginning on page 209.

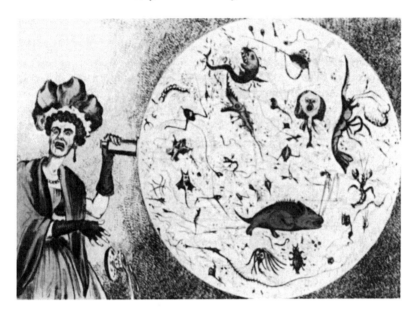

Fig. 2. A caricature on the contents of a drop of water from the Thames River in London, 1828. This etching by William Heath was entitled, "Monster Soup." (Original on file at the National Library of Medicine, Bethesda, Maryland.)

England (Fig. 1), but it still remains debatable whether the standard of living of workers, particularly the industrial and urban poor, was deteriorated or improved by the industrial revolution by 1825.[2] This revolution of iron and steel was associated with increased urban pollution, both in the air and water (Fig. 2). There is no doubt, however, of the rising cost of food and of the squalid living conditions of most rural and urban residents. In England foreign trade problems and occasional poor harvests contributed to wretched economic conditions. Between 1815–1825 a cluster of grievances existed for the British people, including slavery-like factory conditions, unjust criminal codes and landlord difficulties, religious hardships and an unreformed Parliament.

In the new United States of America the Federalist presidents were in office, and a period of relative political stability extended from 1801–1829. Most Americans lived in the country (91.3 percent by 1830), though cities were gaining population on the eastern seaboard. The Napoleonic Wars adversely affected American trade and continued to disrupt American politics (1805), but by 1816 economic conditions improved, and both the American industrial revolution and westward expansion over the Appalachians tended to lift the spirit of nationalism. Both the population and area of the United States doubled from 1800 to 1825, and the Lewis and Clark Expedition initiated by Thomas Jefferson, and the Louisiana Purchase added enormously to this new country.

General Scientific and Technical Background

Along with the industrial revolution, technological advances and practical inventions (Table 2) conjointly increased in the early nineteenth century. The electric carbon arc light (1801), reliable steamship (1807), electric telegraph (1809), steam locomotive (1814), photography (1814), use of gas-lamps in London (1814), and central gas heating (1821), were invented or

Table 2
Discoveries in Chemistry and Physics
and Practical Inventions (1800–1825)

1800   Laplace published *Mécanique Celeste* (1799–1825). Herschel discovered infra-red rays in spectrum.

1801   J.W. Ritter discovered ultra-violet rays in spectrum. Sir Humphry Davy invented electric carbon arc light. *Disquisitiones arithmeticae* by Carl Friedrich Gauss elaborated theory of numbers.

1802   John Dalton stated chemical law of multiple proportions. Thomas Young described wave theory of light.

1804   John Dalton published atomic theory.

1807   Robert Fulton's steamboat, Clermont, in U.S.A. proves economic success and reliability of steamships. William Hyde Woltaston invented camera lucida and suggested stereochemistry. Sir Humphry Davy isolated Ca, Na, K, Mg, S and B.

1809   Electric telegraph invented by Soemmerring.

1810   Process of canning of food patented by N. Appert in France.

1811   Poisson published *Traité de mechanique*, memoir on finite difference. Iodine discovered in sea-weed ashes by Courtois.

1813   Sir Humphry Davy published *Agricultural Chemistry*, first clear description of soil analysis for farmers.

1814   William Charles Wells of South Carolina developed theory of dew and dew-point. Niepce developed photography. Fraunhofer's lines in the solar spectrum discovered.

1814   Steam locomotive invented by Stephenson. London lighted by gas-lamps.

1815   Sir Humphry Davy invented safety lamp for coal-miners. Metronome invented by Maelzel.

1816   Humboldt describes climatology on basis of isothermal lines. Selenium and lithium discovered.

1818   Thénard discovered hydrogen peroxide.

1819   First steamship crossing of Atlantic Ocean.

1820   Oersted announced discovery of magnetic effect of electric current.

1821   Medium pressure hot water heating developed. Natural gas central heating developed in New York. Cauchy published major treatise on algebraic equivalences.

1822   Fourier published treatise on heat, *Théorie analytique de la chaleur*.

1823   Chevallier brothers invent achromatic microscope.

1824   Franklin Institute founded in Philadelphia. Carnot published Second Law of Thermodynamics.

1825   Nobili invented galvanometer. Faraday discovered benzol.

deployed. John Dalton's atomic theory was first published (1804), and Sir Humphrey Davy isolated several elements (1807). The development of chemistry and physics provided tools for taking measurements and increasing knowledge in biology and medicine, and this approach derived from the influence of Newtonian dynamics and mechanistic thinking, which had already become evident in the eighteenth century. Some philosophers, particularly in France, believed that Newton's science could be constructed into a mechanical philosophy,[3] and that man could be analysed as a machine. Others, notably in Germany, followed the philosophy of Kant and Hegel and separated human behavior and other real phenomena from the mechanistic thinking of contemporary early nineteenth century science. The Duncans, writing an introduction to *The Medical and Chirurgical Review* in 1799, stated: "We commence the present volume of our Review under circumstances peculiarly auspicious. At no period of medical history has the pursuit of science been more eagerly followed, or the labours of individuals more successfully exerted. Never have so many important problems been under discussion at one time, and which promise so highly in their solution, to meliorate the condition of mankind."[4] The doctrines of philosopher Friederick W. von Schelling promulgated the concept of the empirical approach to medical and social problems. Some of the concepts followed during the early nineteenth century were completely fallacious, such as phrenology, in which human character and mental capacity were adduced from the conformation of the skull (Fig. 3).

The invention of the voltaic cell in 1800 by Volta, the development of a logical and convenient decimal system for measuring weights and lengths in France (1791–1820), and elucidation of electromagnetic waves helped accelerate general scientific progress at this time. Use of lenses for magnifying small objects had been accomplished since the Middle Ages, and by 1590, the Dutch microscope maker, Zacharias Janssens, had combined lenses to improve their resolving power. Various other later inventors, including Malpighi, Leeuwenhoek, and Hooke further refined the microscope, and by the 1820's improved compound microscopes with achromatic lenses were developed. An illustration of an 1810 model, compound microscope is shown in Figure 4. Though these crude microscopes allowed investigators to observe microcirculation such as capillary blood flow, and individual cells composing tissues or blood, it was still the pre-microbiologic era through 1825; most bacteria were too small to be seen by the early microscopes.

The Milieu for Biology and Medicine

The science of biology began at the dawn of the nineteenth century. The term, "biology" was first noted in the literature in 1800 in a footnote of an obscure German medical publication, and was mentioned in scientific treatises by the German naturalist, Gottfried Treviranus, and the French botanist turned zoologist, Jean Baptiste de Lamarck. By 1820, this new term had gained

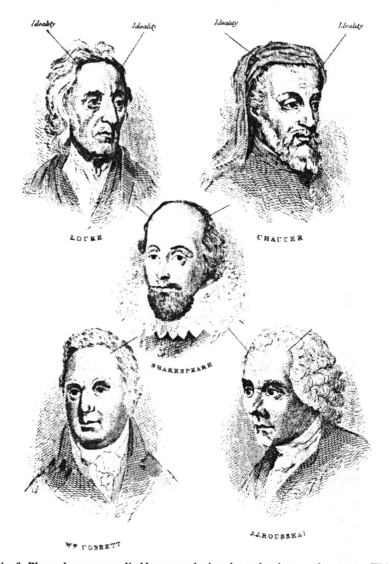

Fig. 3. Phrenology was studied by many during the early nineteenth century. This etching was taken from an early nineteenth century journal devoted solely to this subject.

significant popularity, but it required several more decades in the nineteenth century before biology really developed as a flourishing science. During the first quarter of the nineteenth century, the concept of biology was more limited than today in that it excluded natural history, the description and classification of plants, animals, and minerals, leaving this to the separate domain of the *Naturalists*. Lamarck's definition of biology was

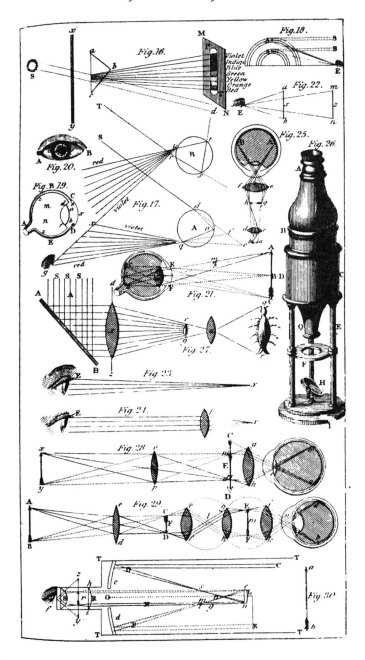

Fig. 4. A compound microscope of 1810. (Taken from an etching in "Letters on Natural and Experimental Philosophy, Chemistry, Anatomy, Physiology, and Other Branches of Science Pertaining to the Material World." Rev. J. Joyce, J. Johnson and Co., St. Paul's Church Yard, London, 1810.

> Biology: this is one of the three divisions of terrestrial physics; it includes all which pertains to living bodies and particularly to their organization, their developmental processes, the structural complexity resulting from prolonged action of vital movements, the tendency to create special organs and to isolate them by focusing activity in a center....[5]

Thus, the earliest domain of "biology" had a functional or physiologic perspective, though it differed from the longer standing field of human physiology (dominated mostly by physicians who occasionally used animals for experimental purposes) because it focused on study of animal and plant function for its own sake. Though Edinburgh and Leiden had earlier been the centers of greatest excellence for medical instruction and life science investigation in Europe, from 1790 to 1840 France was the most prominent center in the West for this activity.

The structural basis for human physiology and biology was, as would be expected, more advanced than correct understanding of function. Francois Magendie, the famous French physiologist, stated in 1816: "We find (physiology) founded upon mere suppositions, to which every one attaches at pleasure the numerous phenomena of life, thinking that he is explaining them satisfactorily."[6] Human anatomy was well developed prior to 1800, and by the conclusion of the eighteenth century the role of tissues, as opposed to organs and organ systems was being elaborated. The French comparative anatomist, Georges Cuvier (1769-1832) developed a scheme of *functional* anatomy. From 1790-1815 Cuvier was the leader of comparative anatomical studies, which were developed to a particularly high level in France.[7,8] Furthermore, in France at this same time, physicians in Parisian hospitals were effecting a revolution in medicine by combining careful postmortem examinations of diseased patients with the clinical descriptions of the patients' disease during life. Xavier Bichat (1771-1802) in France combined the *tissue doctrine* of Cuvier with such clinical-pathophysiological observations of postmortem dissections and published the landmark contributions, *Traité des membranes*, in 1800, and *Anatomie générale* in 1801.

Early nineteenth century physicians had no real knowledge of the means of contagion of disease (though Jenner's experiments on smallpox and cowpox began to elucidate one aspect of this problem), or of the true etiology of most diseases. Thus, their theories on treatment, as delineated throughout the present book, were usually based on erroneous conclusions. Active therapy was the hallmark of medical practice in the early nineteenth century, and those treatments such as bloodletting, purging, cold water dousing, etc., which produced immediate reactions in the patient were thought to be most useful. A form of logical rationalization, usually based upon erroneous conceptions of physiology and disease, was frequently employed by the early nineteenth century physician to justify his mode of therapy. Sometimes the reasoning was based upon experimental observations on human or animal investigations. Increasingly, however, throughout the nineteenth century all forms of therapy

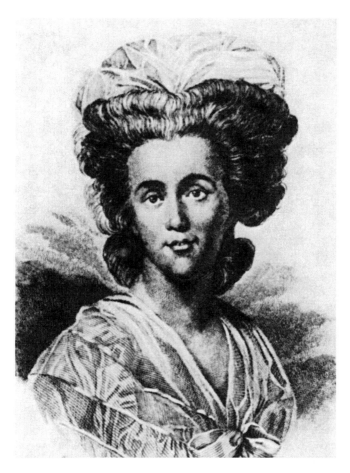

Fig. 5. Madame Necker (Susanne Naaz; 1739–1794). Just before the turn of the century, Madame Necker made notable contributions as a nurse and hospital administrator in Paris.

were to be looked upon with a more critical eye. In the early quarter of the nineteenth century there were also some physicians, laymen, and other critics who thought that any meddling with God's own plan for healing was harmful to the patient. Except for the use of female midwives, a practice which was debated vis-à-vis the superiority of males versus females for this calling, most all physicians were male. Nonetheless, the direct benefit to patients by nurses and other women in the early nineteenth century has been undoubtedly under-rated in most historical treatises. One female health worker who made most notable contributions just prior to the turn of the century was Madame Necker of Paris (Fig. 5). Madame Necker (1739–1794) studied medicine and architecture in order to reform one of the hospitals in Paris. She proved that the best medical

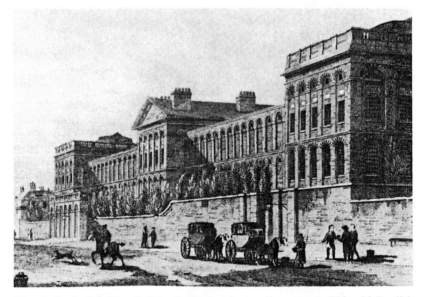

Fig. 6. St. Luke's Hospital in the early nineteenth century. This old English engraving shows that the fine architecture of some of the medical facilities far out-reached the capacity of the service within.

and nursing hospital care, as could be provided in comfortable and relatively sanitary hospitals of that time, was no more expensive than the slovenly care found in other hospitals.

Medical schools, licensing, and societies became greatly increased in number and complexity during the early decades of the nineteenth century, with training both by formal reading and apprenticeship being required, and with considerable variation in training found between city-centers of medical importance (Fig. 6) and rural sparsely-inhabited regions. Further details of this important topic are presented later in the present monograph, and elsewhere.[9] In spite of the increasing attempts for quality control in medical training and the increasing acceptance of "scientific" medicine, dialogue persisted on the values of scientific principles. Examples of this are indicated in the following two selected quotations, by Mr. Tupper and Dr. Buchan, respectively:

> All the truly useful and scientific knowledge we can ever hope to gain, can only be had by observation and experiment; many of very superior intellect have already been so prone to theoretical speculatons as to materially injure the cause which they meant to improve....[10]

and

> The cure of diseases does not depend so much upon scientific principles as many imagine. It is chiefly the result of experience and observation. By

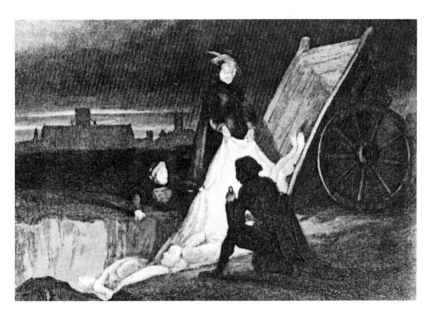

Fig. 7. "The Plague Pit," an engraving by J. Franklin showing a burial scene in the early nineteenth century England. (Original on file at the National Library of Medicine, Bethesda, Maryland.)

attending the sick, and carefully observing the various occurrences in diseases, a great degree of accuracy may be acquired, both in distingishing their symptoms, and in the application of medicines. Hence sensible nurses, and other persons who wait upon the sick, often foresee the patient's fate sooner than many who have been bred to physic [diagnosis]. We do not, however, mean to insinuate that a medical education is of no use: it is doubtless of the greatest importance, but it never can supply the place of observation and experience.[11]

The above technological developments, industrial revolution, and increasing tendency toward the beginnings of a scientific approach to medicine might suggest an increase in optimism toward medical care in the early nineteenth century. Though such pride may have existed in some physicians, it must be recalled that western societies were still subject to the periodic and vicious episodes of plague and epidemics of smallpox, a high toll due to tuberculosis, typhoid and numerous other infectious diseases. As clearly depicted in early nineteenth century etchings (Fig. 7), the public's fear of such diseases was constant. Yearly religious ceremonies in Marseilles, France reminded the inhabitants of the 1720 visitation of the plague. The first cholera outbreak, which began in India in 1817, had reached Britain and France in 1831 and 1832, respectively. Daumier captured the morbid mood of this cholera epidemic (Fig. 8). Rats, which carried bubonic plague through their fleas, were a menace in every city. Professional rat killers offered their services to the public

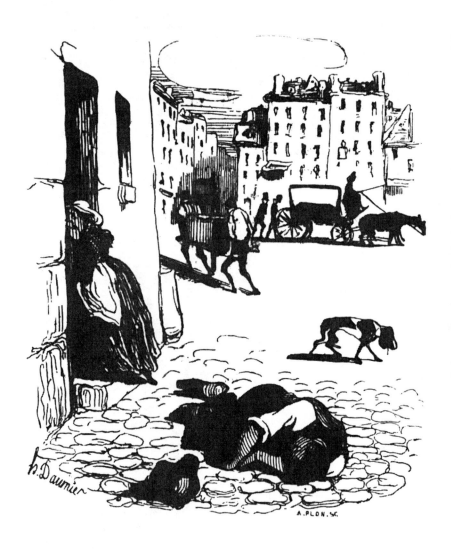

Fig. 8. A wood engraving by Daumier (1841) illustrated the morbid atmosphere during a cholera epidemic. (Original on file at the National Library of Medicine, Bethesda, Maryland.)

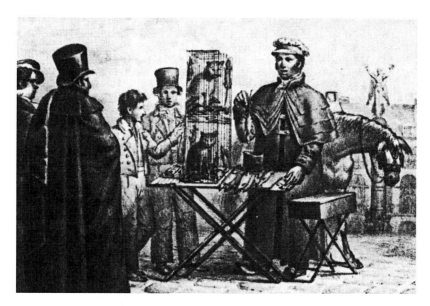

Fig. 9. Street scene of a nineteenth century rat killer offering his services in France. Lithograph by Jean Henri Marlet, entitled, "Le marchand de mort aux rats." Fleas on rats were carriers of bubonic plague. (Original on file at the National Library of Medicine, Bethesda, Maryland.)

(Fig. 9). Thus, against the rising scientific developments in medicine, by 1825 few tangible improvements in reduction in morbidity had been accomplished, with the exception of some reduction in smallpox due to early vaccination schemes. Table 3 summarizes the most notable landmarks in medicine and biology in this period.

Table 3
Landmarks in Biology and Medicine (1800–1825)

1800   *Traité des membranes* published by Xavier Bichat. Royal College of Surgeons of London chartered. Total thyroidectomy for goiter performed by Hedenus. Jennerian vaccination against smallpox introduced in U.S.A. by Waterhouse. First use of word *Biology* in obscure German medical publication. Purification of water by chlorination in France and England (in this pre-microbiologic period). Systemic description and interpretation of fossils began in Paris by Georges Cuvier (extinct vertebrates) and Jean Baptiste de Lamarck (marine shells).

1801   *Anatomie descriptive* and *Recherches sur la vie et la mort* published by Xavier Bichat. Thomas Young first described astigmatism. Pinel published psychiatric treatise. Toulouse Medical Society founded.

1802   Word *Biology* publicized in Germany (Gottfried Treviranus) and France (Jean Baptiste de Lamarck). Health and Morals of Apprentices Act in Britain; protects child and female laborers. Phrenology propounded by Gall. Paris Health Council founded, as important urban public health organization. First Children's Hospital, Hospital des Enfants Malades, founded in Paris.

1803   Société anatomique founded in Paris. Société de pharmacie founded in Paris. Medical Instruction Regulation edict in France. *Medical Ethics* published by Thomas Percival. Hemophilia described by Otto.

1804   Arteriosclerosis described by Scarpa. Philadelphia Medical Museum (journal) founded. Peritonitis described by Laennec. Royal London Ophthalmic Hospital founded. Fever Hospital (House of Recovery) opened at Leeds.

1805   Morphine isolated by Sertürner. Cerebrospinal meningitis described by Vieusseux in Geneva. Polish Society of Physicians founded. Royal Medical and Chirurgical Society of London founded. First Boston Medical Library opened. L. Oken suggested cell theory. Thomas Young stated surface tension theory of capillarity. W. H. Pepys of London introduced amalgam for dental fillings.

1807   Swedish Medical Society founded in Stockholm. College of Physicians and Surgeons founded in New York. College of Medicine, University of Maryland, founded.

1808   Interscapular-thoracic amputation performed by Ralph Cuming.

1809   Ephraim McDowell (Kentucky) initiated abdominal surgery in U.S.A. by successful oophorotomy. Endocarditis described by Allan Burns. J. B. Lamarck, published *Philosophical Zoology*, classification by function rather than structure. Importance of cells in living organisms. Yale Medical School founded.

1810   Typhus and thyphoid fever described by Hildenbrand. Bayle described essential tubercle. Wollaston discovered cystin in calculi. Rheumatism of the heart described by Wells.

1811   Founding and incorporation of Massachusetts General Hospital, Boston. *System of Anatomy* published by Dr. C. Wistar in U.S.A. Spinal nerve-root function discovered by Sir Charles Bell. Neurilemma discovered by Keuffel.

1812   Appendicitis described by Parkinson. Action of vagus on respiration described by Legallois. Academy of Natural Sciences founded in Philadelphia by citizen subscriptions. Bellevue Hospital founded in New York. Beginning of *The New England Journal of Medicine and Surgery and the Collateral Branches of Science*, U.S.A. Benjamin Rush published first American book on psychiatry.

1813   A. P. de Candolle, *Elementary Theory of Botany*. Treatise on Toxicology published by Orfila (1813–1815). Langenbeck excised uterus for prolapse. Robert Watt published treatise on whooping-cough.

1814   *London Medical Repository* founded.

1815   Medico-Chirurgical Society founded in Glasgow. Successful hip-joint amputation by Guthrie. Lipase action discovered by Marcet. Chair of midwifery established at Glasgow University.

1816   Laennec perfects stethoscope, presents major treatise on auscultation. Hamburg Medical Society established.

1817   G. Cuvier, animal kingdom divided into four groups or Embranchements. *Child Mortality*, published by J.B. Davis, recommended preventive medicine and health screening of poor. Medical Society of District of Columbia established in U.S.A. Scleroderma described by Alibert. Rhode Island Medical Society established. Extra-uterine pregnancy described in book by John King.

1818   U.S. Congress passes bill for reorganization of Army staff: Joseph Lovell is first Army physician to be appointed Surgeon General. Innominate artery successfully ligated by Valentine Mott. J.F. Meckel systematizes birth abnormalities. Proust discovered laucin. Cardiac insufficiency described by Corvisant.

1819   Hunterian Society founded in London. Hay fever described by John Bostock. Harvard Medical School Library founded.

1820 Philadelphia *J. of the Med. and Phys. Sciences* founded by Nathaniel Chapman. Académie de médecine founded at Paris. Iodine used in treatment of goiter. Embryology treatise published by Von Baer. First U.S. Pharmacopoeia published.

1821 Philadephia College of Pharmacy founded. Charing Cross Hospital established in London. Veterinary High Schools established in Stockholm and Stuttgart. Société de médecine founded at Rouen. Magendie founded Journal de physiologie experimentale (Paris).

1822 Willaim Beaumont, M.D. acquired patient, Alexis St. Martin in Michigan for classic experiments in gastric physiology. Paris Medical Faculty suppressed. *New Guide to Health* (botanic drugs) published by Samuel Thomson in U.S.A. Experimental hospital gangrene produced by Ollivier by autoinfection. Hysterectomy performed by J.N. Sauter.

1823 *Lancet* founded by Thomas Wakley in London. Flourens demonstrates role of cerebrum by cerebration. Gastric and pancreatic juice described by Tiedemann and Gmelin. Purkinje investigated fingerprints. Società medico-chirurgica founded at Bologna. Royal Veterinary College established in Edinburgh. Compound microscope improved by Amici.

1824 R.J.H. Dutrochet described individuality of cells. Prout investigates gastric juice acidity. Advocation of "progressive differentiation of the mammalian embryo" by Ignay Döllinger.

1825 Germinal vesicle in ovum discovered by Purkinje. Bouilland described and localized aphasia. Tubercular peritonitis described by Andral and Louis. The Quarantine Act (London) obliged quarantine for incoming ships without clear bill of health. National Veterinary School established at Toulouse. Jefferson Medical College established at Philadephia. Fever Hospital in New York City opened.

Chapter II

Galvanism — Electrical Machinery for Medical Disorders

> "In no branch of Philosophy have superstition and the love of the marvellous revelled in greater luxury of variety and absurdity, than in every existing disquisition, observation, and theory of the classes of phenomena called electrical"
> — Sir Richard Phillips, 1820.

Pre-1800 Medical Electricity

By the end of the eighteenth century experimental workers and philosophers in many fields, including medicine, botany, chemistry and physics had become increasingly aware of electrical phenomena both in their natural environment and in animal life. They had developed many theories attesting a similarily between static electricity of inanimate objects, electrical discharges such as lightning and a presumed electric fluid of animal and human life, a "principium vitale" or "elementary fire" essential for life. Prior to 1800 simple methods had been contrived to generate electricity, to measure the intensity of positive or negative charge of electricity, and numerous electrical machines had been invented to electrify humans to help cure a large variety of medical disorders. The German physician, Dr. C.G. Kratzenstein, had apparently been the first experimentalist to use electricity for medical treatments, in 1744.[1] Others, such as J.F. Hartmann of Germany[2] and J.R. Dieman[3] of The Netherlands had also published comprehensive texts on medical electricity prior to 1800. Priestley's three volumes on *Experiments and Observations on Different Kinds of Air*, published in 1774–1777[4] also constituted one of the eighteenth century major works on electrical phenomena.

At this time it was generally held that an electric fluid, which was continually in motion, traversed the living but not deceased body, and that this electric fluid was in equilibrium with electrical energy in the atmosphere, as well as in the earth. It was further believed that bodily motion incited and increased the electric fluid within living objects, and that the friction of circulating blood against vascular walls generated electric fluid. Thus, warmth such as "animal heat" (or "caloric," "elementary fire," or "phlogiston") was thought by some nineteenth century scientists to be the same as or similar to their *electric fluid*. According to Hackmann[5] many controversies on this phenomenon existed before 1800; some believed that changes in atmospheric electricity caused changes in bodily electric fluid and function, whereas others disputed this, observing that electricians who were continually exposed to electricity suffered no ill effects. Dieman[3] proposed that electric fluid only influenced the body when it could not pass freely through pores, and therefore could be trapped inside (excessive fluid causing increased pulse rate or enhanced perspiration) or outside (electrical deficiency) the body.

It was generally accepted in the era just prior to 1800 that electricity exerted its greatest effect upon the nervous system, and calculations were made that demonstrated a similar velocity for transmission of both *electric fluid* and *nervous fluid*.[6] Prior to 1800 physicians believed that electricity could be advantageously employed to treat four types of illness, i.e., diseases caused by an irregular function of the "principles of life," and maladies inducing paralysis. The basis for believing that electrical phenomena could be medically exploited had its roots in the late eighteenth century experiments of Franklin, Galvani, Sulzer, Volta, Valli and Aldini. Benjamin Franklin had described the *electric fluid* that composed lightning. Sulzer had described in a 1773 paper pertaining to his "Theorie der angenehmen und unangenehmer Empfindungen" (i.e., Theory of agreeable and disagreeable sensations), that "when two pieces of metal, one of lead and the other of silver, are joined together so that their edges make one surface, a certain sensation will be produced on applying it to the tongue, which comes near to the taste of martial vitriol, whereas each piece by itself betrays not the least traces of that taste."[7] Later, in 1791–93, Galvani of The Bologna Institute of Sciences reported his initial experiments on animal electricity. His accidental discovery of the influence of electricity on neuromuscular tissue was dependent upon his observant science students.

Whilst Mr. Galvani was dissecting a frog on the table, whereon accidentally stood an electrical machine, one of his pupils happened to touch the nervus cruralis of the frog with the point of the dissecting knife, upon which, immediately, the muscles of all the members were convulsively contracted. Another standing by, thought he observed that this phenomenon took place when a spark was drawn from the conductor of the machine, an idea which was afterwards confirmed; for, on touching the same nerve of another frog, and likewise pricking it in order to assure himself whether it was owing to his having accidentally wounded the nerve, without drawing a spark at the same time, not any motion ensued; but if the nerve was touched with the point of a knife, at the time when he had ordered a spark to be taken from the machine, the same phenomenon appeared again.[7]

The electrical machine used by Galvani was similar to that developed by Volta, the so-called "voltaic pile," which was a pile of discs of different

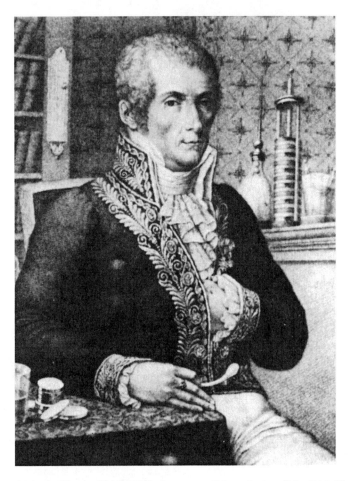

Fig. 10. Volta, of Pavia (1745–1826). Inventor of the voltaic cell in 1800. Note the voltaic pile in the right background.

metals with layers of cloth interposed. Such an apparatus induced an electrical charge which was measured in the late 1700's as positive on one metal and negative on the other. Volta (Fig. 10) and other early experimenters had observed that the power of this charge was increased by wetting the cloth with salt water, and that the induced current could decompose water into its constituents, oxygen and hydrogen. Further, it had been observed and reported, prior to 1800, that the metals became *oxydated* (oxidized) as a result of exposure to this electrical current. Humboldt[8] later showed that "Galvanic contractions" in the frog could be obtained without the intervention of any metal, and he therefore concluded that nerves had a galvanism different from muscles, and that in animals a galvanic fluid continually passed back and forth between nerves and muscles. Geoffrey, Volta and others[8,9,10] also pointed out a similarity between the Galvanic pile (voltaic pile) and the electric organs of the silurus and torpedo fish (currently referred to as the electric eel), the latter which contained a series of parallel, hexagonal prisms filled with a soft transparent substance. Humboldt's experiments were later refuted in 1801 by Pfaff of Kiel[11] who stated that, "after having read his work, we are but little more advanced in the physiology of organized bodies than we were before." Pfaff thought, wisely, that "we ought rather to confess our ignorance of the unknown process of vitality, than content ourselves with a hypothesis so completely imaginary as M. Humboldt's." Then, not so wisely, Pfaff continued, Humboldt "conceives that such an application of chemistry to the physiology of the human body, impedes rather than advances our progress in science. We go to rest in an agreeable dream; we think we know and we cease to inquire."

General Concept of Galvanic Principles and Electricity, 1800–1825

Although it was not until later in the nineteenth century, when Faraday (1821–54) and Maxwell (1865) worked out the main theories of electricity and electromagnetism, the earlier theory of Franklin was accepted by many but not all in the early nineteenth century. Martin Van Marum of the Netherlands was one such supporter of Franklin's theory, according to which "all electrical phenomena are explained by the nonequilibrium of a single fluid called the electric fluid."[12] Van Marum, who had earlier constructed the famous Teylerian electrical machine in 1784, propounded this *single* electrical fluid theory through 1819. Others, such as Du Fay, Symmer, and Coulomb in France advanced the theory that there were two distinct fluids producing the two opposite electrical forces, *positive* and *negative*. The positive electrical force was referred to as the "vitreous electric matter," and the negative, the "resinous electric matter." By studying the physical shape of electrical charges (analogous to mini-lightening bolts) produced by the electrical machine, and observing the reverse direction of such bolt patterns under reversed charge conditions, Van Marum confirmed his belief in a single electric fluid.[12] John Cuthbertson, Philosophical Instrument Maker and Fellow of the Philosophical Societies of Holland and Utrecht also supported Franklin's theory.[13]

The Rev. William Jones of Northamptonshire and Suffolk was a natural philosopher who published comments on electricity in 1800, also with views toward Franklin's theory. Jones presented a discourse on the distinction of materials that allowed passage and dissipation of electricity which he termed, *conductors*, and *nonconductors*. He further described two types of electricity, an *effluvium* which could be emitted wholly by glass, and a new force which he termed, *reverberatory*. His account[14] of the reverberatory electrical force is noteworthy:

> Muschenbroek had suspended a glass vial of water at his conductor, and was electrifying it to try how long the water enclosed by the glass would retain its electricity: but, in doing this, he grasped the bottle with one hand

to remove it, while, his other hand touched the conductor; and in this instant he received a stroke through his arms and breast, attended with such a sensation as no man had ever felt before, and which he that has once felt will never forget. This was a wonderful fact; and soon as Muschenbroek had made himself master of it, he reported it. The fame and the practice of it soon flew into every civilized part of the world. People of both sexes, and of all ages and conditions, repaired in crowds to see and receive this wonderful shock; and the public curiosity was so much awakened, that every body was ready to hear what writers had to say upon the subject. Dr. Watson, a physician, gained great reputation by his manner of treating it, and I heard several learned persons pronounce his work to be the best that appeared upon the occasion. He made no scruple to call the new power of electricity by the name of *elementary fire*, and his electrical machine a *fire-pump*.

The Rev. Jones, who was not opposed to fusing his scientific philosophy with his religious or political feelings, spoke further of the identity of lightning and electricity. He commented that

which of the two was first in bringing down fire from the heaven; whether Romas of France, or Franklin of America, has not been well ascertained, so far as I have been able to learn; but let it be Dr. Franklin; for them the fact will be an ominous prelude to the business he was soon afterwards to do in the world, in drawing down the fire of civil war upon his country, and spreading the confusion of anarchy over the earth. The Frenchman may certainly put in his claim; for the omen will agree as well with his present national character: but we need not trouble ourselves in settling their respective shares: they have it all between them; there being no others who have so just a title as the American and the Frenchman to be called the incendiaries of the world.[14]

This quotation was atypically political for *The London Medical Review*, in part perhaps because its originator was a minister rather than a doctor. It was published during the Napoleonic wars with France, seven years prior to the beginning of seizure of U.S. ships by Great Britain, and eleven years prior to declaration of war against Britain by the American Congress.

Debate on Equality of Electricity and Galvanic Fluid

Increased experimentation with the voltaic or galvanic pile after 1800 naturally resulted in controversial interpretations of the theoretical basis electrical phenomena. Dr. John Bostock presented his theory of action of the galvanic apparatus in 1802.[15] He provided three postulates:

First, that the electric fluid is always liberated or generated when a metal or any oxidable substance is united to oxygen; secondly, that the electric has a strong attraction for hydrogen; and thirdly, that when the electric fluid, in passing along a chain of conductors, leaves an oxidable substance to be conveyed through water, it unites itself to hydrogen, from which it is again disengaged when it returns to the oxidable conductor.

An indentity of electric and galvanic fluids was allegedly proven by M. Carlisle in a commentary of *The Medical and Chirurgical Review* in 1800.[16] Carlisle found that

> a number of plates of silver, as forty or fifty (crowns or half crowns) piled alternately with plates of zinc, having pieces or melted pasteboard between each to complete the galvanic chain, will not only give an electric shock to the person who touches the top and bottom of the series, but will continue to give an uninterrupted stream of the electric fluid; which being passed through water decomposes it completely. If gold, silver, or platina wire, be employed to carry the electric matter into and from the water, both oxygen and hydrogen are liberated; but if oxidable metals are employed, hydrogen only is procured.

Another comment in the same journal noted that

> a more calm investigation of the subject, however, has shown that the phenomena of galvanism are by no means referable to a peculiar property residing in living bodies, but that these are acted upon by the galvanic influence, as by a stimulus merely; and there seems, in fact, little reason to doubt, that this *influence* is one and the same with that of the *electric fluid.*[17]

Duncan and Duncan, of Edinburgh, interpreted Humboldt's opinion of galvanic phenomena,[18] i.e., "What issues out of the nerves seems to act upon them as a stimulus when it returns into them." and "... The phenomenon of turgescence, or muscular contraction, may be considered as the consequence of a chemical change of mixture, as the consequence of the power of attraction acting without hindrance." It was believed that galvanic fluid was a principal agent in the vital process of each organ, and at any selected point in time, a greater or lesser unequal distribution of galvanism existed in nerve or muscle. The Duncans stated that Humboldt used the term, *galvanic fluid*, for convenience, but that he concluded "its nature, as well as that of caloric (heat), light, electricity, and magnetism, hitherto perfectly unknown."[18] Others, such as Robertson in France,[19] rejected the notion that the *electric fluid* was the active principal of galvanic phenomena. An editorial in *The Medical and Chirurgical Review* proposed the following question.[20]

> Finding that chemical attraction is destroyed, increased, and diminished, according to the galvo-electrical states of bodies; and as all bodies which unite chemically seem to be in opposite states of electrical energy, the question is proposed, — Whether chemical unions and disunions are not occasioned by the varying states of these energies; or whether chemical attraction is not the same thing as electrical energy?

A difference between electricity and galvanism was also described (1807) by Vassali Eandi.[21] A summary of his idea is that there exists naturally a compound fluid, made up of the electric, galvanic, and magnetic fluids, with the matter of heat or caloric, and perhaps light; and that one or the other of these becomes apparent, according to the different bodies which put it in motion, and the variety of their action: that these component parts are present in different proportions, having different affinities for different bodies, and for one another; so that they always tend to unite together to the point of saturation, which forms the natural fluid.

Dr. Philip Wilson, writing in the *Annals of Philosophy* (1816) and in the *Quarterly Journal of Science and Arts* (1820) concluded that the *nervous influence* and *galvanism* were the same.[22,23] By modern standards such a view is still upheld. Indeed, neurotransmission can today accurately be shown to be propagated by a spike potential reflecting a rapidly moving wave of negativity. Interestingly, early nineteenth century workers were partially correct in assessing (or guessing) this phenomenon, as shown in the 1802 statement in the *Medical and Physical Journal*,[24] viz.,

Animals are endued with a peculiar electricity, to which he (Galvani) gives the appellation of *animal electricity*, and which he thinks to be contained in most animal parts, chiefly however manifesting itself in the muscles and nerves. It seems to be secerned in the brain from the blood, whence it is communicated through the nerves to the different parts of the body, but it appears to reside chiefly in the muscles. A muscular fibre is similar to a Leyden phial, and the nerve represents the conductor of the phial, and consequently the whole substance is to be considered as a number of Leyden phials. The external surface of the muscle possesses negative, the internal substance positive electricity. The interior of the nerves is composed of a matter capable of conducting electricity, while the exterior prevents by the oily coating its effusion and dispersion. Muscular motions proceed, when the electric fluid is conducted from the interior of the muscle into the nerve, whence it is brought back again to the muscles, either through the external fluid of the nerves, or through the membranes and the adjacent parts, as it were through an arch — so that, according to the laws of equilibrium, the same quantity may be united in the negative electric part of the muscular fibre, which issued by means of the stimulus in the nerves from the positive electrical part.[24]

Wilkinson, lecturer on galvanism at Soho Square, London attested in his 1804 book[25] on the theory of galvanism that galvanism differed from common electricity

in mode only; the former consisting in the evolution of electricity from conducting bodies, forming one of their constituent parts, and disengaged by a chemical process; while the latter is the same principle rendered apparent to our senses by the temporary change of nonconducting bodies to a conducting state.

Further, he concluded that all the operations of electricity were reducible to the actions and reactions between air and the electric fluid.

The distinguished Robert Hare, M.D., who was professor of chemistry in the Medical Department of the University of Pennsylvania, America's first school of medicine, also studied galvanism.[26] He considered that "the principle extricated by the voltaic pile was a compound of caloric and electricity, both being original and collateral products of galvanic action. In this period Hare contributed many papers, dealing not only with galvanism, but concerned with construction of diverse types of apparatus for chemical experiments. He distinguished *caloric* and *electricity*, suggesting that the former energy permeated "all matter more or less, though with very different degrees of facility." *Electricity*, on the other hand, did not radiate in or through any matter, but did rapidly pervade metals.

In Berlin Dr. Grapengiesser differentiated between elasticity and galvanism.[27] He conducted a series of experiments on different animal species, on himself, and on several of his friends. His conclusion was that galvanism (generated by a galvanic battery) seemed to penetrate more easily and deeper into the nerves, which seemed to be optimal conductors, than electricity. Grapengiesser stated that galvanism was never conducted through dry skin, but that electricity was uniformly communicated throughout the whole animal body, particularly over the surface. Other distinctions were made on these electrical phenomena as well. Wilson, who identified the *nervous influence* with *galvanism*, believed that the vital principle of animal life was not to be confused with galvanism. He stated,

> whether the vital principle be something superadded to bodies, or only a peculiar arrangement of their constituent parts, the fact is, that it bestows on matter certain properties. It is essential that our expression should convey this fact, and no more. The galvanic experiments which have been laid before the reader go far to prove, that galvanism has nothing in common with this principle, because these experiments exhibit them acting parts in the animal economy wholly of a different nature,

and

> it would appear from these observations, that the nervous influence, or galvanism, in exciting the muscular fibre, as in the formation of the secreted fluids, and the evolution of caloric from the blood, operates by effecting a chemical change. Thus, the phenomena of the nervous power seem to be only another field in which galvanism exhibits those striking chemical powers which we have seen it display in other instances.[28]

Berzelius described an interesting, handy way to make the distinction between positive and negative electricity. They

> may be readily distinguished by the taste, on making the electric current pass by means of a point on to the tongue. The taste of the positive electricity is acid, that of the negative electricity is more caustic and, as it were, alkaline.[29]

Writers, even in the early nineteenth century, realized the dilemma of theorizing about such electrical phenomena, as did Sir Richard Phillips who suggested

> The philosophical electrician talks flippantly of his fluids and his fires — his negatives and his positives — his charges, surcharges, and discharges — his saturations and nonsaturations — his attractions and repulsions — and other conjurations — and believes that he can bottle up his fluid, *sui genesis*; that a cloud can be surcharged with it; that bodies contain more or less than their natural quantity; and a hundred other equal errors.[30]

Types of Galvanic Apparatus and Electrical Machines

A variety of devices were created in the early 1800's for generating electrical currents and sparks, for measuring the electrical potential, and for electrifying human patients. The design basis of these devices depended generally upon the creations of the electrical piles and tubes earlier invented by Volta, Galvani and others.

A typical generator of electricity was described in 1800.[31] It consisted of alternate series of plates of zinc, silver and wetted pasteboard.

> Mr. Nicholson, having observed a disengagement of gas to take place around the conducting wire, and which seemed to have the smell of hydrogen when the wire of communication was steel, he proposed to ascertain whether it were really so, by breaking the circuit, by the substitution of a tube of water between two wires. Accordingly, a brass wire through each of two cords was inserted at the opposite ends of a glass tube about half an inch in diameter, filled between the corks with water: the distance between the points of the wires in the water, was about an inch and three quarters. This compound discharge was applied so that the external ends of its wire were in contact with the two extreme plates of a pile of 36 half crowns with the correspondent pieces of zinc and pasteboard. A fine stream of minute bubbles immediately began to flow from the point of the lower wire in the tube, which communicated with the silver, and the opposite point of the upper wire became tarnished, first deep orange, and then black. On reversing the tube, the gas came from the other point....

The editor writing the above account noted that when the tincture of litmus was used in the tube instead of water, it changed to a red color, showing that acid was formed. In Holland, Dutch three florin pieces were used for the silver plates instead of British crown pieces. Van Marum and Pfaff in Holland used a pile of 200 pairs of metals to generate a charge on jars. The discharge of the jar produced a 5/8 inch divergence of gold leaves in an electrometer. As a less objective way to measure the intensity of the discharge, these Dutch workers tested the effort on humans[32]:

> With 20 pairs of metals, the passage of electricity was sensibly felt in both

hands, each being wetted, and grasping a copper conductor of two inches diameter. Sixty pairs affected the elbows. With 200, strong shocks were received, extending to the shoulders.

Bolton, of Birmingham, constructed a galvanic pile of 1500 pairs of plates, and one constructed at the French National Institute was able to heat iron wire red hot and vaporize it.[33] Professor Hare of the United States described his "galvanic deflagrator" and "electrical plate" machines in some detail.[34,35] His deflagrator is illustrated in Figure 11. Hare attempted to quantitatively relate the *chemical effect*, i.e., the amount of gas generated, with respect to the number of plates in the galvanic pile. The maximal chemical action was not reached with 2000 plates, and he postulated that at least 4000 to 6000 plates would be required for a maximal effect. In contrast, *spark generation* was maximal with 600–800 plates, and diminished with additional plates.[26]

Details of construction of several types of galvanic apparati were published in the early 1800's. One type, described above with pasteboard and metallic plates, was described in 1801 in modified form.

> If pieces of polished tin, about an inch square, and 1/20 inch thick, be connected with woollen cloth of the same size (moistened, some in water, and some in diluted nitrous acid), in the following order, tin, acid, water, and so on, till twenty series are put together, a feeble galvanic battery will be formed, capable of acting weakly on the organs of sense....[36]

A more powerful class of galvanic batteries was constructed of single metals with fluids, when metallic substances which were "oxidable in acids, and capable of acting on solutions of sulphurets, were connected as plates."[36] If zinc and copper plates of large area were used with a conductor liquid of one part sulfuric acid, one part nitric acid, and 60 parts water, a large current was achieved, as described by Oersted.[37] Colonel Haldane found the following combinations of metal, of decreasing order of power[17]:

zinc — with gold, silver, iron, copper, lead, tin, mercury

iron — with mercury, gold, silver, copper, lead, tin

lead — with gold, silver, copper, tin, mercury

tin — with gold, silver, copper, tin, mercury

copper — with gold, silver, mercury

silver — with gold

Several types of galvanic batteries are illustrated in Figure 12, including the submerged plate type and the vertical glass column containing metallic coins. One type with submerged vertical plates consisted of

> twenty copper and twenty zinc plates, about 19 inches square ... supported vertically in a frame, the different metals alternating at one half inch distance from each other. All the plates of the same kind of metal were soldered to a common slip, so that each set of homogeneous plates formed one continuous metallic superficies. When the copper and zinc surfaces thus formed are united by an intervening wire, and the whole immersed in an acid, or aceto-saline solution, in a vessel devoid of partitions, the wire be-

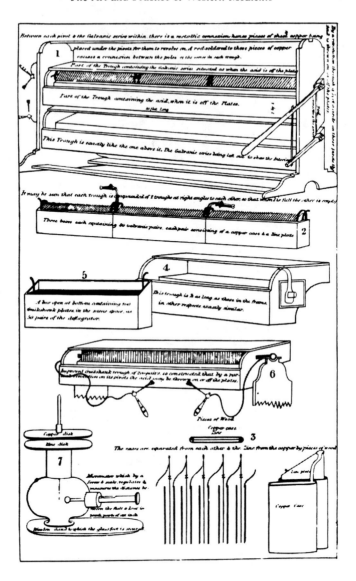

Fig. 11. Professor Hare's single leaf electrometer and improved deflagrator (1824).[34,35]

comes intensely ignited; and when hydrogen is liberated, it usually takes fire, producing a very beautiful undulating or corruscating flame.[26]

Professor Davy of Bristol lectured at the Royal Institute of Great Brittain on the history and principles of galvanism. He presented details of his 500 plate "grand galvanic battery," shown in Figure 13.[38]

ELECTRICITY and VOLTAISM.

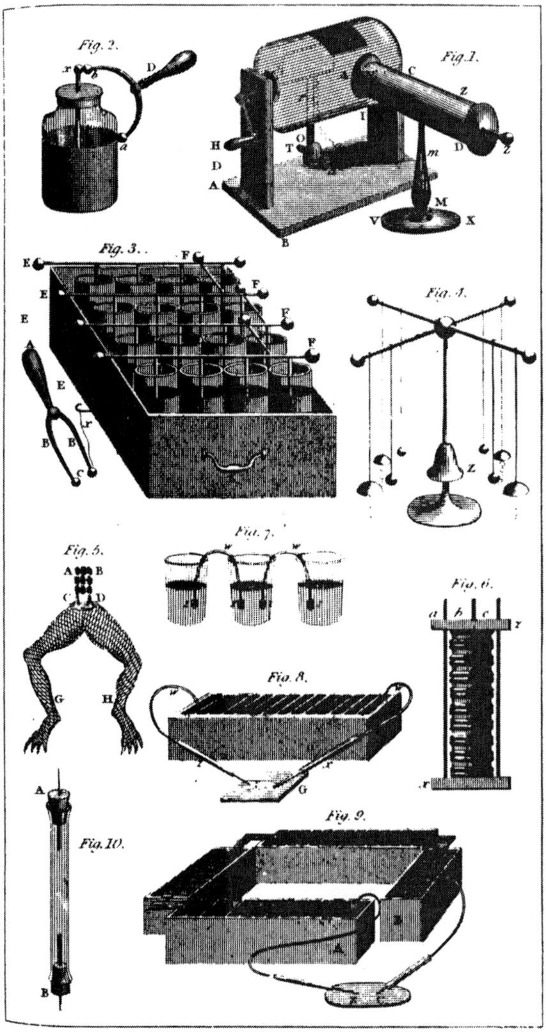

Fig. 12. Several types of galvanic batteries used in 1810. (Etching taken from Joyce, Rev. J., "Letters on Natural and Experimental Philosophy, Chemistry, Anatomy, Physiology and Other Branches of Science Pertaining to the Material World," J. Johnson and Co., St. Paul's Church Yard, London, 1810, p. 306.)

The electrolytic decomposition of water was commonly observed after use of the plate galvanic pile. A method for conveniently collecting the resulting gases was described in the *Medical and Physical Journal* in 1801, after the method of Cruikshank.[39] It was reiterated

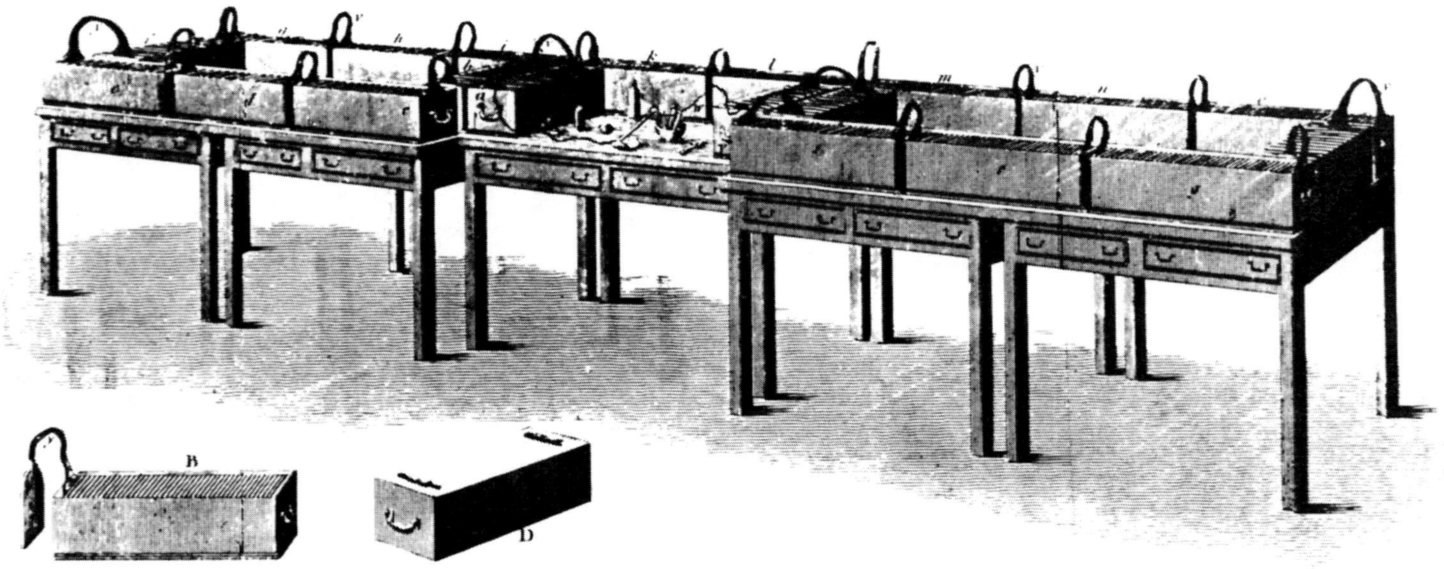

Fig. 13. Professor Davy's 500 plate "grand galvanic battery," 1808[38]

in order to procure these two gases separate from each other, to estimate their quantities, and examine their nature more particularly, Mr. Cruikshank took a glass tube, ten inches in length, and by means of a blow-pipe bent it in the middle until the legs formed an acute angle, resembling the letter V. While the glass was red-hot, he contrived to blow an opening at the angle, about one-tenth of an inch, or a little more, in diameter. Two gold wires, passed through corks secured by cement, were introduced into the legs, and brought within an inch of each other at the bend: the tube was then filled with distilled water, and a finger placed on the opening at the angle, to prevent the fluid from escaping. It was placed in a tea-cup containing water, with the angle downwards, the legs having an inclination of about forty-five degrees. The extremities of the wires being then brought into contact with those of the pile, a quantity of gas was disengaged from both; but by far the most from that connected with the silver. By this contrivance, the gases from the two wires were obtained perfectly distinct, each gas ascending in the leg of the tube which contained its generating wire. On examining the gases, that from the wire connected with the silver end of the pile was almost pure hydrogen, and that from the zinc end almost pure oxygen, in the proportion of two parts by measure of the former to one of the latter, or nearly in the proportion in which they exist in water.

Not all medical writers agreed that water was composed as was correctly stated by the above investigator. One correspondent to *The Philosophical Magazine* in 1800 stated,

> If a particle of water is composed of a particle of oxygen and a particle of hydrogen, what rapid currents must be of those two substances! Where the oxygen is produced, the hydrogen must first descend to the bottom of the leg of the syphon, pass through it, and appear at the wire in the other glass, and vice versa with the oxygen.[40]

The inverted glass syphon, attached to a galvanic column containing 400 square inches of zinc and 400 of copper was also used by Dr. Moyes of Edinburgh.[41] Moyes reported that "when the syphon was filled with a purple infusion of red cabbage, everything else remaining the same, the liquor or fluid in one leg soon became red, and that in the other as soon became green." Dr. Moyes concluded from his experiments in 1800 that water "was not decomposed by furnishing gas to the galvanic influence; it giving no oxygen where it furnishes hydrogen, and no hydrogen where it furnishes oxygen." Thus, we can again observe an oft repeated fallacy of early nineteenth century medicine: logical but incorrect conclusions based upon gross, empirical observations. Such misjudgments simply resulted from a dearth of correct theoretical knowledge. Arsenious acid was similarly subjected to decomposition in the glass syphon by influence of the galvanic pile, by both Moyes[41] and others,[42] who observed deposition of metallic arsenic on the one electrode.

Dr. Hare devised a single gold-leaf electrometer, consisting of a glass vessel, ball, and gold leaf which responded to charges of electricity induced in the apparatus. As a device to measure electricity, it would "not be expected (to work) in weather unfavourable to electricity."[29] Several German experimenters advanced the design of galvanic piles, consisting of gold and zinc or silver and copper metals separated by cloth moistened with salt water, by terminating one of the conductors in a fine pointed wire iron, and the other in a knob.[43]

The electrolyte solutions (conducting liquids) or moist materials in electric piles were tested for efficiency. It was observed that pure starch or starch impregnated with different salts,[44] concentrated sulphuric and nitric acids,[45] acetic acid,[46] and moist pasteboard sufficed. Dr. Heidman of Vienna tested[47] over 50 different conducting liquids, including saliva, egg whites, etc., and reported that muriatic acid and oxymuriatic acids were optimal for galvanic actions.

Galvanic devices for medical purposes typically consisted of voltaic piles and attached electrodes, such as illustrated in Figures 14–16. A commentary in *The Medico-Chirurgical Journal and Review* of 1816 stated that

> the most convenient apparatus for medico-electrical purposes consists of a circular glass plate, measuring from 18 to 28 inches in diameter, and revolving between two pairs of dry leathern cushions, a conductor, Leyden jar with a moderately sized cylinder, and medical electrometer. With a machine thus constructed, and its appurtenances, an insulating stool or chair, a brass ball or wooden-pointed director mounted in glass and having a wooden handle, another director inserted in wood, and some small wire or chain, electricity may be applied to the human body in a variety of ways, so as to be augmented or diminished in every possible degree, and to correspond with every curative intention.[48]

The electrical charge was popularly applied to the ear while the patient wore a specially made headdress, such as the one shown in Figure 15. A large array of conducting electrodes was designed, as illustrated in Figure 17.

Galvanic Experiments on Animals, Blood, and Deceased Criminals

In the early nineteenth century many experimenters tested the effects of electricity, generated by galvanic piles, on living and dead animals. Professor John Aldini of Bologna was one such investigator.

> Being desirous to examine, according to the principles of Galvani, the power of an arc of animal moisture in warm-blooded animals, I recollected that I had several times observed simultaneous convulsions produced by these means in two frogs, and recently in the heads of two oxen, the arc being conveyed from the one to the other in different ways. I placed the two heads in a straight line on a table, in such a manner that the sections of the neck were brought into communication merely by the animal fluids. When thus arranged, I formed an arc from the pile to the right ear of one head, and to the left ear of the other, and saw with astonishment the two heads make horrid grimaces; so that the spectators, who had no suspicion of such a result, were actually frightened. It was, however, observed, that the convulsions excited in the heads disposed in this manner were not so strong as

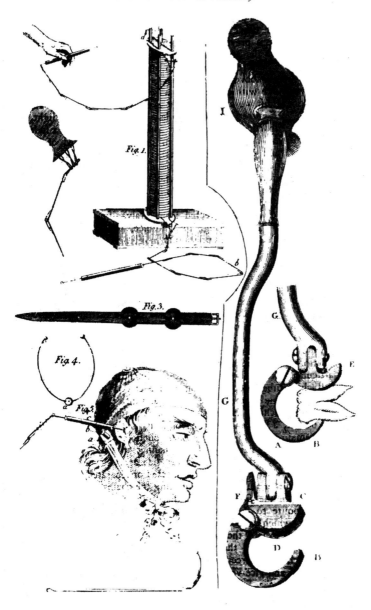

Fig. 14. Medical applications of the galvanic apparatus (early nineteenth century etching). (Ref. 62, 1802)

those produced when I performed the experiment on each head separately. It is certain that, in this experiment, the arc of animal moisture supplies the place of a continuation of the nervous and muscular fibres.[49]

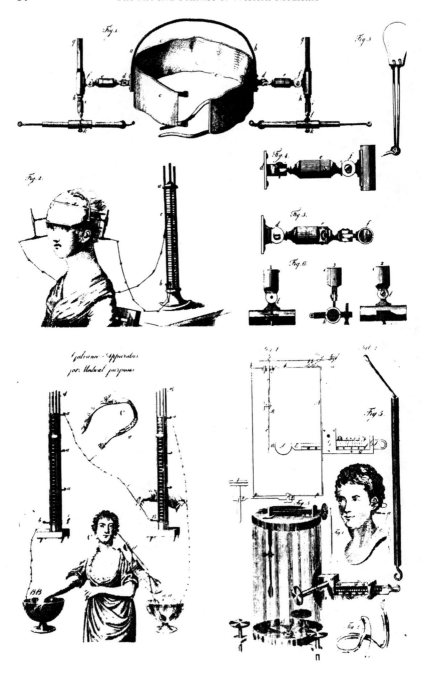

Top: Fig. 15. Details of the headdress, attached to a voltaic pile (1816) Ref. 48. Bottom: Fig. 16. Medical galvanic apparati of Dr. Bischoff, 1802. Engraving taken from "Medical and Physical Journal," 7 (1802) 528–40.

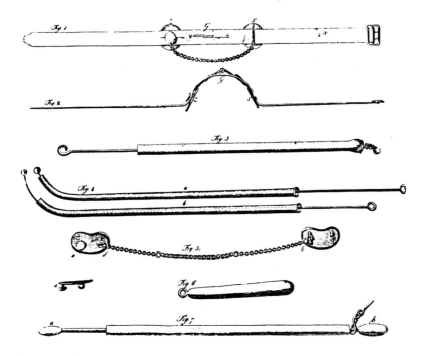

Fig. 17. Conducting electrodes employed in the medical application of galvanism. (Early nineteenth century etching.) (Ref. 63, 1803).

This investigator further reported many experiments upon the exposed brain of the ox, forming arcs with the optic nerves, eyelids, lips and eyes.

Other experimenters found that the heart of the dead frog remained excitable for much longer (15 hours) than that of a decapitated human (4½ hours), after stimulation by the galvanic pile.[50] Further, Dr. Thomson of Edinburgh constructed a galvanic apparatus from animal tissues. He recorded[51]:

> After trying every experiment mentioned in most systems of animal magnetism, I made a pile of thin slices of brain and muscle, which, by a single piece of metal, produced the most violent agitation in a frog. It even produced a slight effect without metal.

The Royal Academy of Sciences at Berlin offered in 1820 a 300 ducat prize, to be awarded to the best essay on animal magnetism.[52]

Antivivisectionists had their origin early in medical history, and some of them criticised the use of animals in medical experiments. Dr. Wilson Philip was criticized for his use of animals in experiments of galvanism. However, the editor of *The Medico-Chirurgical Journal* came to his rescue[53] in 1818, stating,

> We are, indeed, sick of that maukish sensibility that sheds a flood of crocodile tears over the corpse of a rabbit, put to death for the purpose of

pathological or physiological research, while it can behold, unmoved, hecatombs of animals every day sacrificed to satiate the appetite of sensuality and gluttony. Let us look around us, and we shall see one half of Nature slaughtering and devouring the other half. Is it not meritorious, instead of censurable, to inflict death on a small animal for the purpose of lessening human suffering, or prolonging human life?[53]

Because blood was considered in the early nineteenth century to be a *vital fluid* which contained the very substance of life, and that the natural galvanic properties of tissues and organs also reflected a *vital* property or *galvanic* fluid, experiments were performed applying exogenous galvanism to blood. Professor Tourdes of Strasburgh communicated in 1801 to Professor Volta[54]:

The confidence and friendship of which you have so often given me proofs during my residence in Italy, embolden me to communicate to you the result of an experiment which appears to me to resolve one of the most disputed points of physiology, that of the vitality of the blood. This liquid deprived of the serum, lymph, etc., reduced to the fibrous part, and subjected to your galvanic or rather electric apparatus, (for the identity of the galvanic and electric fluids have been established in an incontestable manner by your late researches) at the temperature of about 30 degrees of Reaumur, exhibited a trembling oscillation and palpitation analogous to those experienced by flesh of animals newly killed; a double motion of contraction and dilatation, sensible to the eye by means of a magnifying glass; a characteristic mark of the vital force peculiar to the muscles, cellular tissue, etc.

Other reactions of blood to the galvanic influence were reported in 1802. Delametherie of France found that "when any portion of clotted blood adhered to the fibrine, and was touched by the conductor from the top of the pile, its colour, which before was of a dark hue, changed instantly to a pale-red colour."[50] Today, since we know that oxyhemoglobin is red and hemoglobin is bluish, we might theorize that oxygen, formed electrolytically from water in the blood clot, oxidized the reduced hemoglobin observed by the Delametherie and caused this color change. It is likely that this experiment has never been repeated during the past 150 years! Delametherie observed that the color change took place only if the positive electrode of the pile touched the blood clot, and concluded therefore that oxygen was responsible for the color change.

Dr. Caldwell also studied the effects of galvanism on blood, which was considered to be "possessed of life."[55] He confirmed that galvanized blood coagulated faster than control, nongalvanized blood from healthy human subjects. Further, he attempted to prove that a very strong galvanic shock to blood might prevent its coagulability, since "the blood of animals that are destroyed by lightning will not coagulate." He demonstrated this to a limited degree with blood drawn from a young healthy gentleman, and concluded that the electrical current had caused "the partial extinction of life" from the blood. Everard Home also galvanized blood, while attempting to study the physiology of animal secretions. He noted[56] that electrical power can separate albumen from blood, and also observed the color change induced by galvanism as described above.

Newly deceased human subjects were employed in early experiments with galvanism, both for the purposes of studying the scientific relationship of animal electricity with respect to life, but also with the hope that useful galvanic therapy could be developed for revival of asphyxiated or paralyzed patients. Mr. Crewe, according to Dr. Augustin's 1802 account, suggested stimulating the brachial nerve of unconscious subjects with the galvanic power; if convulsions ensued, it could be concluded that the patient was alive, with incitability left in the body, but if "no commotions are produced by the strongest Volta's pile, a total want of vital power must be supposed."[57] Kelch, of Königsburg undertook galvanic experiments on the body of a criminal who was beheaded for a capital crime. Immediately after execution he placed the head upon a table and stimulated it with a pile of sixty-two plates of zinc and copper. He was able to induce the opening of the victims eyes, contraction of the upper lip, undulation of the tongue, and a motion similar to the act of swallowing.[58] John Aldine, professor of experimental philosophy at the University of Bologna, acquired considerable reputation for his galvanic experiments on the body of a malefactor executed in 1803, as well as on patients deceased following "putrid fevers, by pleurisies, by wounds in the pericardium, by the scurvy, and by the consequences of parturition."[49] By immersing the hand of an unconscious patient in a solution of muriate of soda, and establishing a current arc, Aldini induced contractions of different degrees in the hand and arm, "the importance of this method for determining the duration of the vital powers after death ... (were) readily comprehended."[49] Professor Aldini noted, upon stimulation of the head of a criminal, after creating an arc from the mouth to the ear, that

> the jaw immediately began to quiver, the adjoining muscles were horribly contorted, and the left eye actually opened ... (and) on applying the conductors to the ear and to the rectum, such violent contractions were excited, as almost to give the appearance of reanimation.[59]

During his residence in England Professor Aldini exhibited galvanic experiments at Oxford, at Mr. Wilson's Anatomical Theatre in London, and at St. Thomas's and Guy's Hospitals. The grateful lecturers and pupils of these two hospitals presented him with a gold medal, "in honourable testimony of their approbation."[60]

Medical Uses of Galvanism

In Western Europe and in the British Isles, galvanism had gained increased but still questioned popularity for the treatment of a variety of medical ailments by the early nineteenth century. Diseases treated by this mode of therapy ranged from blindness, deafness, paralysis, and asphyxia, to pain, hydrophobia, urinary calculi, and insanity. We can judge today that, in spite of the general optimistic acclaim for this treatment by most medical writers in 1800–1825, galvanism would have had 1) either no real beneficial effect, 2) a positive influence due to psychologic placebo action (which in part accounts for the continuance of patient acceptability of treatment, most often by quacks, by fake electrical machines in some regions of the world even today), or 3) a temporary positive action simply by overstimulation of some impaired function in an organ system. This is not to imply that modern medical science has established complete knowledge about interactions between biologic function or malfunction and exogenous electrical energy. Indeed, in somewhat rare instances modern experiments are still being conducted to show interesting and possible benefits of electrical energy in very selected situations, such as promotion of wound healing or bone repair.

In the early nineteenth century galvanism was also known to be potentially dangerous, when employed for medical therapy. Dr. Anthony Mongiardini, a member of the Italian National Institute, stated in 1807 that[61] "Galvanism disposes bodies to putrefaction. Muscular fibres, blood, urine and bile, when galvanized, became putrid sooner than the same substances not galvanized." Further, Dr. Augustin, of Berlin, commented in 1802,[62] that

> In employing it [galvanism], however, for the cure of diseases we should always consider the topical as well as the general state of irritability, in order to prevent any bad consequences which may arise by applying too strong a degree of this stimulus. A strong galvanic shock generally occasions lassitude and a kind of lameness, which continues for a whole day, particularly if we have for any long time exposed ourselves to the action of the battery. Thus, Mr. Rutter, a gentleman to whose ingenious experiments we are particularly indebted for many interesting explanations with respect to this subject, felt a general indisposition attended with weariness and dullness in the head, after having exposed himself for a whole hour to the action of a strong battery, which consisted of 100 strata. Inflammations of the eyes after continued experiments with light, debilitated insensibility of the tongue, catarrhs after frequent experiments in the nose, vertigo and head ach after violent strokes through the head, and tooth-ach, which always ensue after any experiment being for some time continued at any of the above parts of the head, are the common consequences of galvanising, which undoubtedly arise from this stimulus having acted too violently on the sound degree of irritability.

Deafness was one of the principal diseases treated by galvanism. Known to arise from various causes, deafness was only recommended for treatment by galvanism if it was thought to be caused by paralysis of the acoustic nerve, or if the secretion of ear wax to be promoted.[62] Grapengiesser of Berlin published details in 1803 on the application of galvanism for diseases of the auditory organ, delineating five different methods. For "the application of the simple galvanic chain on wounds, occasioned by blisters behind the ears," he recommended[63]

> A blister being applied behind each ear, a plate of silver, and another of zinc, are put on the two places which have been deprived of their epidermis, after which they are connected by means of a gold and silver chain; the first of which appears to increase the efficacy of the apparatus. The whole is preserved in its proper situation by a head bandage. The apparatus shows itself particularly efficacious, when the zinc plate lies close to the place, while the silver plate is rather loosely fastened, that it may be alternately pressed to the wound, and removed from it. On pressing this plate close to the wound, the appearance of lightning and a gentle tinkling in the ear will be perceived. The time during which this apparatus is suffered to act, depends on the incitability of the patient, and similar circumstances. In general, I found eight to ten, and sometimes only five hours to be sufficient for producing some effect.

Mr. Strenger of Iver administered

> the galvanic influence, in a case of deafness, by applying a small ball to the external orifice of the ear; while a much larger one (was) held in the patient's hand; the communication (was) then formed and interrupted alternately by means of machinery, once in every second, for about four minutes daily, for two or three weeks.[64]

He asserted that he thus restored the sense of hearing to forty-five persons.

Galvanism was applied to deaf and dumb patients at Kiel, with temporary and slight improvement in hearing of some patients, allegedly by producing "merely a momentary irritation on the nerves of hearing, during the time that it (was) ... employed; and that this irritation (was) ... followed by weakness or relaxation of the parts."[65] This finding was also reported in Stockholm.[66] Mr. Frischsen, a Benedictine and professor of philosophy at Salzburg successfully "cured" a number of deaf patients by means of a galvanic pile consisting of 300 plates.[67]

As would be predicted, the application of galvanic shock would tend to exert paramount influences on neurological and sensory functions, such as described above for deafness. Convulsive diseases, such as epilepsy, were often considered as candidate diseases for therapy by galvanic powers. Dr. John Whittam in Germany,[68] and Whittam in Nottingham[69] used it for treatment of epilepsy. According to Mansford in 1819,[70]

> Epilepsy has ever been a disease so extraordinary and frightful in its appearance; so obscure in its nature; and so rebellious to treatment, that the Ancients attributed it to the anger of the Gods. Hippocrates, indeed, endeavoured to combat this idea, but still applied to it the appellation of *Morbus Sacer*. Like as in phthisis, cancer, and some other opprobria medicorum, the *successful* — nay the *infallible* methods of treating epilepsy, would fill a volume; yet, in a great majority of instances, it still defies the physician's skill, and preserves a headstrong course towards the destruction both of the mental and corporeal functions.

Nonetheless, Mansford continued that galvanism offered a most suitable mode of therapy for epilepsy.

Galvanism was also employed for general paralysis in England[71] and France,[72] for hemiplegia,[73] and for asphyxia.[73,74] It was used for relief of hoarseness, as described by Dr. Augustin of Berlin.[62] An 1813 case history in this regard, described by Parker Cleaveland, Esq., professor of mathematics and natural philosophy in Bowdoin College in the new United States of America[75] is illustrative:

> At first I permitted him (the patient, Mr. P., who could speak only in an imperfect whisper) to receive several shocks from a Leyden jar, of the capacity of one pint, about half charged, causing the fluid to pass from one hand to the other through the arms and breast. This charge he did not appear to feel above the wrists. I then gave the jar very nearly its full charge, and passed it two or three times through the breast. He then spoke, in a very audible manner, saying "my voice is coming." His voice then resembled that of a man somewhat hoarse with a cold. He added, "I feel a little of it (meaning the numbness) yet about the lower part of my breast." I then passed two or three similar charges through the part in which the numbness was felt. By this time, Mr. P. spoke with his natural voice, and, as he assured me, with perfect ease; being entirely free from any numbness. As he was leaving the laboratory, I observed that the finger which he had applied to the brass knob of the jar, was entirely devoid of colour. It was cold and incapable of sensation. I passed a few charges through it, and in the course of a few minutes its colour returned.[75]*

"In cases of mania, or raving madness, the application (of galvanism) was found to be hurtful, and even dangerous," according to Aldini in 1803.[49] For pain, such as from sciatic nerve neuralgia[76] and back pain,[77] it was considered effective. Hydrophobia in patients, caused by the bite of rabid animals, was reported to be cured by galvanism in 1804.[78] Patients with chronic rheumatism were afforded "great relief"[79] or "temporary relief"[80] by galvanism.

According to Dr. Martens in 1803, the rationale for employing galvanism for rheumatic complaints was that it "diminished activity of the cutaneous organ, suppressed transpiration, or any other obstruction in the cutaneous vessels and the tela cellulosa, etc."[81] Dr. Bischoff also described the use of galvanism for arthritic disease.[82]

The extraction of urinary calculi from the bladder was reportedly facilitated by galvanism, in 1824.[83] The Swiss physiologists, Prevost and Dumas, also demonstrated in dog experiments that a small fusible calculus, when brought between the conductors of a galvanic battery, underwent gradual decomposition within the bladder.[83] In women with paralysis of the sphincter vesical urinariae, the following procedure was recommended:

*Note that this source of current was the Leyden jar, rather than the galvanic pile; some writers in this era made the distinction between galvanic versus electrical fluid. Note also that the experimenter was professor of mathematics rather than a physician. This general interest in medical effects of galvanism is also apparent in reference 77 by Richard Teed, a jeweller at Lancaster Court, Strand.

The zinc conductor is brought into the intestinum rectum, while the conductor of the silver side is applied above the arcus ossium pubis, on the moistened skin, or on a wound made by a blister, or the first conductor may be immediately applied to the collum vesicae through the vagina.[63]

Thus, as a final note on the supposed virtures of galvanism for medical therapy, the philosophic comment of William Hutchins, in 1803, is noteworthy:

Actual experiments, and the facts resulting therefrom, being the only certain means of arriving at a knowledge of the operations of Nature, whether as to their causes, effects, combinations, affinities, or other attendant phenomena, it is of the utmost importance that all deductions drawn from them should be stated, and transmitted to the public with precision and accuracy....[84]

Chapter III

The Medicinal Leech
as a Blood-letting Agent

In the early history of medicine few therapeutic agents or procedures were accepted with such confidence or were practiced as extensively as blood-letting. Amongst the various procedures in Western medicine found suitable for this purpose, the employment of leeches ranks high in historic interest. The use of leeches was popular from the early days of the Roman Empire during the reign of Augustus, through the Middle Ages and Renaissance, and finally reached an era of greatest popularity during the first quarter of the nineteenth century. Even today, in an era of antibiotics, open heart surgery, and organ transplantation, the use of leeches is occasionally, though rarely, encountered. However, current use of leeches is restricted to the cosmetic removal of superficial, subcutaneous hemorrhage from local regions.

During the early nineteenth century (1800–1825) an atmosphere prevailed which facilitated the natural propagation of those therapeutic techniques which were held in high esteem. This was the period of the Industrial Revolution—first in England and later in continental Europe, of the French Revolution (1789–1815) and the rise and downfall of Napoleon (1800–1815), and subsequently of the Congress of Vienna (1815) and the age of Metternick (1815–1830). The Napoleonic victories were followed by a flourishing period in both the arts and the sciences, most notably and early in France, but subsequently also in the rest of Europe, England, and the new United States. In France, Marie François Xavier Bichat founded the discipline of histology with his *Anatomie Générale* (4 vols., 1801), *Traité d'anatomie descriptive* (5 vols., 1801–3), and other treatises. Dr. F.J.V. Broussais (1772–1838), one of Bichat's students began to dominate, in France the medical scene with his doctrine of "physiological medicine," in which he emphasized that disorders of function were more influential than disorders of structure. In this light, it was felt that the vital phenomena of the human body depended upon external stimuli such as heat or other environmental agents, and that the physician should attempt to dominate nature and its external stimuli. Broussais felt that all diseases were local and were related either by transference via sympathetic means or by means of the gastrointestinal mucosa. All excessive stimuli resulted in hyperemia and inflammation, and the basis of all pathology was gastroenteritis. Hence, a perusual of the French medical literature of this era readily reveals the widespread acceptance of Broussais' therapeutic philosophy. This philosophy recommended the alteration of the external or internal (gastroenterologic) stimuli by use of purgatives, blisters, stimulants, or other agents, and by blood-letting through venesection or the application of leeches to the stomach or head with the hope of curing or preventing gastroenteritis. Though many of these modes of therapy were also in widespread use in the British Isles and elsewhere in Europe, Broussais himself (Fig. 18) was not widely acclaimed in countries other than France.

The General Philosophy of Blood-Letting

It is difficult to establish the geographic location where blood-letting was first practiced. Hippocrates rarely prescribed this procedure, but physicians of Cnidian origin (a Lacedemonian colony in Asiatic Doris) frequently practiced blood-letting during the Fourth Century B.C.[1] Later during the Second Century B.C., Greek physicians serving in Rome commonly employed blood-letting, as did the Jewish physicians during the Fifth Century A.D. During the late Middle Ages blood-letting was the usual treatment for plethora, a morbid condition thought to be due to an excess of blood in the body. The directions for phlebotomy, or venesection during this era were very specific, and were almost always determined by astrological considerations. The philosophy behind blood-letting during this time was the shunting of morbific material from one organ to another, or the removal of excess blood. By drawing blood from one side of the body opposite to where the malady was, it was thought that the disease was directed to the unaffected organs where it might better be controlled. Alternatively, when bleeding was attempted on the same side as the disease site, it was felt that it would diminish the plethora and relieve pain.

In the first quarter of the nineteenth century general blood-letting was employed in cases of inflammation, pain, spasm, etc. with the hope of removing plethora, congestion, and pain as described by the Broussais school. The efficacy of copious local bleeding was vigorously propounded by the Briton, Vaidy[2]:

> General blood-letting has often failed in general diseases, from the timid manner in which it was employed; and there is great reason to believe that local blood-letting, in local diseases, especially those termed *spasmodic*, has not been carried to an extent sufficient to insure success, in numerous instances. Our continental brethren employ this kind of evacuation much more frequently, and perhaps much more successfully than we do; therefore, we shall be wise in taking a lesson and a hint from our rivals ...

Another author[3] purported the efficacy of blood-letting by various means for the cure "of fever, endemic, and contagious; more expressly the contagious fever of jails, ships, and hospitals, (and) the concentrated endemic ... yellow fever of the West Indies." Hence, blood-letting was recommended "in the commencement of fever, whether the disease declares itself by the symptoms of a paroxysm, violent, and in form, or only by headach, and general uneasiness," and one author[3] was in the habit, "particularly in time of sickness, and in subjects lately arrived from Europe, to order blood to be drawn from the arm to the amount of twenty ounces, or upward." Other authors[4] relied upon blood-letting for the treatment of gout (Fig. 19) believing that it "diminished pain, prevented congestion or effusion in the more important organs, (and that it prevented) ... the premature wearing out of the system by the violence of the attacks." A Scottish physician[5] during the first quarter of the nineteenth century concluded, in a book devoted to the efficacy of blood-letting (*A Practical Treatise on the Efficacy of Blood-letting in the Epidemic Fever of Edinburgh*), that blood-letting calms respiration, improves the appetite, checks nausea and vomiting, removes coma or delirium, prolongs life, cuts short epidemic fever, retains diarrhea, alters the type of fever "to one more favorable," etc. (Fig. 20).

Statistics from the House of Recovery and Fever Hospital in London for the year 1810 reveal that 209 patients were "blooded" for various fevers according to the following numbers: cephalic fever, 45 (cases); hepatic fever, 34; pulmonic fever, 31; enteric fever, 22; gastric fever, 15; cardiac fever, 11; peritoneal fever, 3; remittent fever, 5; and mixed fever, 43. Since the death rate of those patients subjected to blood-letting in this hospital was less than 4.5 percent, the hospital official reported in a manner typical of the didacticism of the era:

> We are not afraid of any mischief resulting from its [blood-letting] sudden adoption. The well-informed practitioner, who thinks for himself, will weigh its merits by his own previous observations and experience, before acting upon it; while the man of mere routine, will jog on as usual, until roused, by the reiterated success of others to venture on its application.[6]

The Leech in Historical Perspective

Most of the historical writings indicate that the leech was used as one of several tools of bleeding throughout most of the history of blood-letting as described above. The leech, called βδελλκ by the Greeks, *Hirudo* by the ancient Romans, *Sanguisca* by the modern Italians, *Sangsue* by the French, *Blutegel* by the Germans, *Blodigle* by the Danes, and *Pijavuka* by the Poles, is described in historical perspective in several monographs of the early Nineteenth Century. Vitet's book, *Of the Medicinal Leech*[7], published in France in 1810, Thomas' book, *Memoire pour servir a l'historie naturelle des sangsues*[7], published in France in 1806,

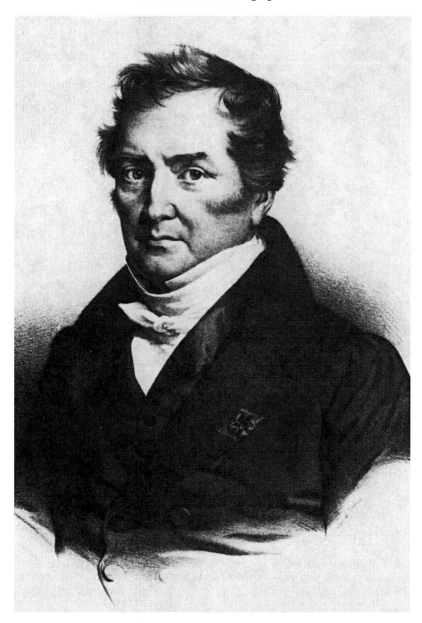

Fig. 18. Dr. François-Joseph-Victor Broussais (1772–1838) graduated in medicine in 1803 and served as military surgeon for Napoleon. A promoter of the concept of organs as a site of disease, and that life depends upon heat and irritation, Broussais considered that gastroenteritis was the basis of all pathology. His doctrine of copious blood-letting undoubtedly contributed to many deaths. (Original on file at the National Library of Medicine, Bethesda, Maryland).

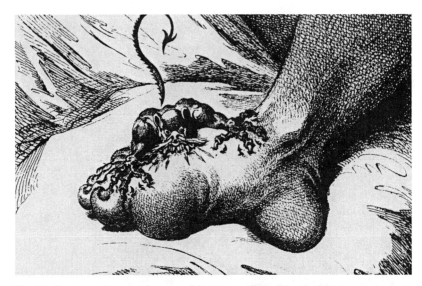

Fig. 19. Gout was frequently treated by the medicinal leech. The beast shown in this well-known 1799 etching is not, however, a leech. This etching entitled, "The Gout," was by the Englishman, James Gillray, who was a celebrated political caricaturist. This medical caricature depicts the four cardinal signs of inflammation earlier described by the Roman physician, Celsus; pain, fever, redness, and swelling. The original of this etching was colored.

and Johnson's book, *A Treatise on the Medicinal Leech, Including its Medical and Natural History, with a Description of its Anatomical Structure; also, Remarks upon the Diseases, Preservation, and Management of Leeches*, published in London in 1816[8] all describe the historical background of the leech. Suffice it to say here that its use was popular along with other external "cures" such as venesection, cupping, blistering, scarification, caustication, cauterization, and other procedures. Themison, during the first years of the Christian era, used leeches along with cupping glasses. During the fourth century Oribasius wrote of the advantages of leeches, and Aretaeus recommended leeches in the treatment of angina when the patient feared the lancet. Pliny, Zacutus Lusitanus, Horatius Augenius, Aetius, and many other less notable physicians wrote of the efficacy of leeches.

The rapid growth of medical practice, inquiry, and documentation that was omnipresent in Western Europe and Great Britain during 1800–1825 was accompanied by expanded popularity in the use of leeches as agents in bloodletting. The high regard of this animal is well illustrated in the tone of the following editorial footnote which accompanied a case history in the 1819–20 issue of *The Medico-Chirurgical Journal* of London[9]:

> It is a humiliating circumstance to perceive that some medical practitioners of reputed talent and experience, in the nineteenth century, are denouncing topical bleeding as useless and unnecessary. If the understandings of such

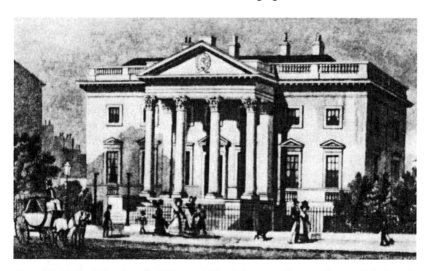

Fig. 20. Hall of the Royal College of Physicians on George Street, Edinburgh, Scotland, from 1775-1843.

practitioners be not under the absolute dominion of prejudice and erroneous reasoning, to the total preclusion of conviction, an instructive lesson would be afforded them by a dispassionate reference to Johnson's *Influence of Tropical Climates*, or *The Atmosphere of the British Isles*; to Parry's *Elements of Pathology*; or to Yeats on *Hychencephalus*. Either of these valuable productions would clearly exhibit the fallacy of their doctrines, and would set their judgments right, on a highly important point of practice. — Editors: *The Medico-Chirurgical Journal and Review* 2 (1819-20) 141.

During the period 1800-1825 leeches were used to such a great extent that they became scarce, particularly in the British Isles. One physician[10] reported that leeches were very plentiful in Aberdeen around 1798, being brought by hawkers from Musselburgh and Edinburgh and sold to apothecary shops for nine to ten shillings per hundred. However, around 1805-1816 leeches became quite scarce. Johnson[8] claimed that England depended upon foreign and precarious sources; imported leeches were principally supplied from Bordeaux and Lisbon. He further stated that "we employ at least one hundred foreign leeches for every English one," and that "many persons are excluded, by its consequent high price, from the benefits of the operation, or purchase them by sacrifices and privations which, in the time of sickness, they are but ill prepared to sustain."

The Therapeutic Use of Leeches

By the early nineteenth century leeches were advocated for ailments too numerous to list here in entirety. However, the following maladies, as indicated by Vaidy[2] in 1819, give some perspective to the almost universal application of these beasts. Toothache (twelve leeches applied to the jaw), gout (thirty leeches applied around the knee), acute rheumatism (twenty leeches applied to each limb), chronic pleurisy (thirty leeches applied to the chest), facial muscular spasm (fifteen leeches applied to the spasm), and chronic pulmonitis (thirty leeches applied to chest) were all treated by local blood-letting. Dancer[11] reported the efficacy of blood-letting in yellow fever if the remedy was applied during the earliest stages of the disease. Beddoes[12] further stated (in faithful allegiance to the Broussais school) that in all types of fever blood-letting by means of applying "relays of dozens" of leeches, supplemented by intermediate subtepid fomentations upon the abdomen, was the recommended therapy, since the fever surely related to the inflammatory disposition of the abdominal viscera. Similarly, French workers[13] prescribed the external application of leeches for gastroenteritis associated with "cerebral phenomena," or for strangulated inguinal hernia.[14] The general association of plethora with inflammation, which was the basis for blood-letting, is typified by the following quotation from Dihmar[15] in the 1823 *Annales de la Médecine Physiologique*:

> N'est-il pas de toute évidence pour des yeux non prévenus, que i'inflammation dont convient le rapportem était due a une pléthore generale bien prononcée, et si palpable, que des taches sanguines l'annoncaient d'une manière incontestable?

Occasionally, special cures were attributed to blood-letting by leeches in the early nineteenth century. Notably, the immediate relief of fits in children, due to "some mischief in the brain," was purportedly the result of leeches applied to the temples of the children.[16] Another report of successful treatment of inflammation of the eye, based upon 2074 cases, was published by Crampton in 1822.[17] This London physician applied leeches directly to the conjunctiva, and not surprisingly noted a much greater unloading of the turgid vessels of the conjunctiva than when the leeches were applied to the temple and eyelids. Dr. Crampton presented great detail for the application of leeches, including the application of leeches to inflamed tonsils after securing the leech by a thread passed through the tail. Another surgeon, Mr. Kentish from Newcastle-upon-Tyne, reported in 1800 the marked and rapid reduction of inflammation at an amputation stump resulting from the application of leeches to the local inflammation, accompanied by venesection in another limb.[18]

A rather divergent viewpoint on the mechanism of blood-letting was expressed by the Londoner, Yelloly[18] in 1819 in the *Medico-Chirurgical Transactions*. He felt that the benefits of blood-letting were not limited to the removal of inflammation, but that other effects were produced in the body, particularly in the nervous system. However, the "state of pathological knowledge (was) ... not qualified to account" for the mechanism at that time. In any case, the use of leeches for blood-letting was held in high regard, for when a description of a substitute for leeches was published in 1815 the substitute, a modified cupping-glass, was considered with disdain:

> There seems something vulgar in the appearance of such an operation (use of cupping-glass), but it may be convenient, whenever we wish to draw blood from a confined part, or a part not perfectly even in its surface. —J. Welsh: *The London Medical and Physical Journal*, 34 (1815) 64.

The Problems Arising from Leech Therapy

Along with the numerous salutory remarks concerning leech therapy during the early nineteenth century, a few reports appeared delineating the problems that occasionally arose following their use. Although accounts[21] appeared which attributed death to the introduction of "morbid poisons" by the lancet in blood-letting (in this pre-microbiologic era!), cases of excessive blood-letting[21] were associated with patient death,[5] particularly when the blood-letting was performed during terminal stages of sickness. Generally, however, the main problem of leech therapy related to excessive bleeding following the removal of leeches from the patients. This hazard was thought to relate to both the punctures induced by the teeth of the leech, and to an "active congestion of blood from all the neighbouring vessels towards the wounded part."[22] The anticoagulant, hirudin, now known to be manufactured by the leech, was not recognized in the early 1800's. The recommendation was made to apply gum arabic, tinder, or pressure, or to insert threads of twisted lint,[22] sponges dipped in liquid pitch, or powders of aloes, or bole armeniac[8] into the hemorrhagic wound.

Another problematical situation arising from the use of leeches was the inadvertent escape of leeches into the throat or stomach. In this case cold water held in the mouth, or the application of vinegar, garlic, salt water, asafoetida, mustard, or other acrid substances was recommended. One of the classic cases[8] of the time (1816) was the ingestion of muddy water contaminated by a small species of leech, by the French army in Egypt. The mechanical removal of the swollen leeches posed a major problem to the military surgeons.

A general review of the injurious effects of leeches was reported by Dr. James Stuart in 1808[23] in the *Medical and Physical Journal* of London. Stuart concluded that unfortunate consequences resulted from the application of leeches 1) in an inflammatory diathesis before general bleedings were performed, 2) when the patient was in a general gangrenous condition, 3) when the patient was in an extremely "irritable habit," or 4) when the leeches were applied directly to a part affected with inflammation, ulceration, or gangrene.

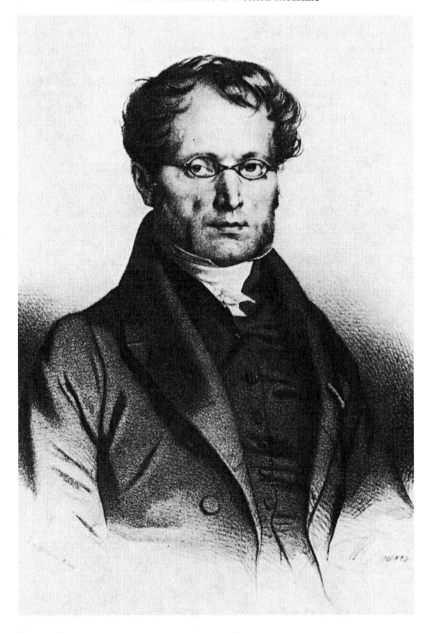

Fig. 21. Pierre-Charles-Alexandre Louis (1787–1872). Louis was the founder of medical (as opposed to vital) statistics, and defined typhoid fever (1829) and phthisis (1825), the latter which was based upon 1,960 clinical cases and 358 dissections. His statistical evidence proved the lack of value of blood-letting as propounded earlier by Broussais (Original print on file at the National Library of Medicine, Bethesda, Md.).

The Maintenance of the Medicinal Leech

Inasmuch as the medicinal leech was extensively employed for blood-letting, the scarcity of the animal required its maintenance in the apothecary shops and physicians' homes so that they could be available on demand, and reused for subsequent bleedings. Thus, various articles appear in the journals of this era which guided the physicians in both the natural history and maintenance of the leech. Large stone vessels equipped with water and marsh horsetail (*equisetum pallustic*), and placed in an area free from unpleasant smells were recommended as storage containers.[8] Cool environments in the summer (60°) and warm environments in the winter (50°) were suggested,[24] as well as pure spring water rather than contaminated river water (as was the case with the Thames River water) for the ideal environment.[25]

The capacity of any one leech to draw blood seldom exceeded one ounce. Hence, relays of 20–30 leeches were applied, as described above, or means were taken to increase the work load of single animals. In the latter case, the tails were cut off the leech in order to provide an unlimited capacity,[26,27] the inflated animals were removed and manually disgorged,[8] or a small amount of muriatic salt was placed at the leech's mouth to induce evacuation.[28] All of these methods were criticized during this period, since the trauma of the procedures resulted in a high mortality of the valuable species. Mr. Bishop, in a letter to the Editors of the *Medical and Physical Journal* stated in 1806[29]:

> I would strongly recommend to you readers and other medical men, the following simple method of treating leeches, and am convinced, from many years of experience, of the great advantage that will accrue from it, particularly as they are become so very scarce and dear. Immediately on leeches falling from a part to which they have been applied, I immerse them in water as warm as new milk, where they are to remain an hour; they are afterwards to be treated in the common way, observing to change the water every second day, they should not be returned to the old stock for at least a week. No means should be made use of to induce the leech to eject the blood it has imbibed. I am preparing a place for the purpose of breeding leeches; should I be successful, I will inform you.

In the foregoing paragraphs an attempt has been made to depict the status of the leech as an agent in blood-letting during the early nineteenth century, an era when this practice reached its greatest prevalence. The utilization of the leech for therapeutic purposes is perhaps a good parameter with which to evaluate the status of medical practice and knowledge during the early 1800's, since it intimately relates to the Broussais concept of disease in general. It is of interest to note that, on the basis of present medical knowledge, most of the cures so adamantly attributed to leeches, by the most prominent medical practitioners of the early nineteenth century, can be assumed to have been the result of spontaneous recovery not related to the leech. Perhaps herein lies a lesson for the modern medical profession! In any case, the devoted intent of the physicians and the developing inquisitiveness of the general medical profession during the pre-microbiologic 1800's is to be admired. Fortunately, the use of leeches probably resulted in less harm than many other procedures which were or could have been practiced in the early nineteenth century. Except for cases where relays of leeches were used, the total amount of blood lost by this practice was probably not significant, and the introduction of infection by this means was probably not too great when compared with venesection, and surgical practices of the day. The benefits of such therapy, if any, were probably related to psychosomatic relief, and perhaps occasional relief of localized congestion or stasis when the leeches were placed upon a localized, superficial region of congestion.

Chapter IV

Concepts and Misconceptions in Cardiovascular Physiology

Historical Precedent and Functional Anatomy

In modern times the cardiovascular system, blood, its circulation, and components are of recognizable paramount importance; we understand cardiovascular physiology well and know that most deaths in developed countries relate to disorders of this system. The perspective of this organ system was rather different in the early nineteenth century. It was indeed recognized as an important, vital system, and was considered medically and pathologically significant, but for all of the wrong reasons. The conveyence of respiratory gases and dietarily derived nutrients, and heat transfer by circulating blood were recognized in this early era. Nonetheless, the relationship of the blood vascular system to the lymphatic system, the true mechanisms of blood flow, the gross basis of cardiac ischemia and some other vascular diseases, the role of the cardiovascular system in the transfer of hormones and immunologic factors, etc., were all unknown in the early nineteenth century. Furthermore, the misconception by physicians of this era, misplacing a great importance on central vascular congestion (especially of the gastrointestinal tract but for other sites as well) as a basis for many diseases resulted in enthusiastic and harmful blood-letting.

From the time of the earliest medical physiologists, the vascular system was considered an anatomic means of transporting vital animal spirits or materials. By 1628 Harvey had published his famous treatise on circulation, *De motu cordis*, a work which had been preceded by his earlier (1618) description of the heart as a bellows-type of pump which maintained pressure in the vessels, and of valves that mechanically directed the flow of the fluid.[1] Up to 1800, no major changes in that concept had occurred. An illustration of Harvey's 1618 translated writing summarizes his view:

From the structure of the heart, it is clear that the blood is constantly carried through the lungs into the aorta as by two clacks of a water bellows to rayse water. By (application of) a bandage (to the arm) it is clear that there is a

> transit of the blood from arteries into veins, wherefore the beat of the heart produced a perpetual circular motion of the blood. Is this for the purpose of nourishment, or more for the conservation of the blood and the parts by the distribution of heat; and, in turn, is the blood cooled by warming the parts made warm (again) by the heat?[1]

By 1800 Harvey's general concepts were accepted by most but not all medical writers. For example, the well-known Dr. C.H. Parry had stated in 1816, "Modern physiology may boast an advantage over the ancient, inasmuch as it has been fully ascertained, that, although the arteries may not be without their spirits, they certainly do convey blood."[2] Still, by 1816 a book was published in Edinburgh by Dr. George Kerr, "professedly against the circulation of blood." His antiquated viewpoint was, however, contrary to the mainstream of physiologic thought in 1816. Part of his rationale was based on the premise that if the ancients were so outstanding or superior in literature, oratory, art, history, architecture, etc., why not in science also? Kerr's views were mentioned in the *Medico-Chirurgical Journal* by Dr. Ewing because he felt that not only should the popular and accepted views be published, "but (it was appropriate) also to take occasional notice of the off-sets or eddies that whimsically play about its (the mainstream) edges, and those frothy bubbles that rise to whirl, and burst, and sink again on its rippling surface." For his aberrant views denying the circulation of blood, Kerr was accused of "nibbling at established doctrines, and his present attempt to eat through the bottom plank in the theory and practice of our art—namely, the Harveian discovery of the circulation."[3]

One example of the level of sophistication and incorrectness of the gross anatomy of the cirulatory system that had been achieved by the turn of the century is shown in Figure 22, showing the anatomy of the heart and of the peripheral vascular system. As described by Dr. James Carson of Liverpool in 1824,[4]

> the general agents which are employed in the circulation of the blood, and which themselves constitute a part of the animal machine, are the lungs, the heart, the arteries, and the veins. There are other agents which may be called general, but which do not peculiarly belong to the animal fabric. The chief of these are atmospherical pressure and gravity. But, in addition to those, there are other powers of contrivances which may be called subsidiary, and of which the office is confined to particular parts of the circulation; among these may be ranked the machinery of the liver and the spleen.

Note that Dr. Carson correctly named the anatomic parts, with the exception of the all-important capillaries, but was physiologically incorrect by overemphasizing the role atmospherical pressure and not mentioning muscular movement, etc. Carson further outlined the functional anatomy of the cardiovascular system, as envisioned in 1824, indicating a high degree of accuracy:

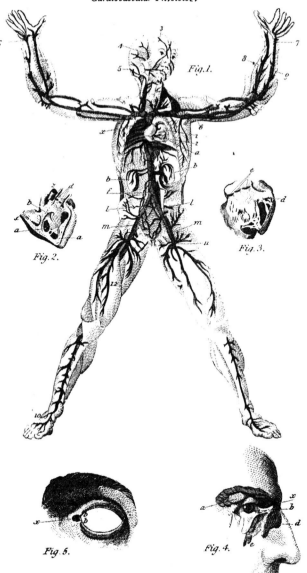

Fig. 22. Early nineteenth century anatomists and physiologists considered the circulatory system to consist of cone shaped tubes, with the base toward the heart, on both the arterial and venous sides. Etching taken from an 1810 British scientific monograph.[19]

Mammalia, and birds having a double circulation, have two hearts included in one, enveloped by a membrane, called the pericardium, — each consisting of an auricle and ventricle, consequently the human heart has four chambers, a right auricle and ventricle, and a left auricle and ventricle;

the two former are actively subservient to the pulmonary or the lesser circulation, and the two latter to the corporeal or greater circulation. There are valves placed between the ventricles and auricles, which favour the passage of the blood from the auricles to the ventricles, but prevent its return from the ventricles to the auricles. The movement of the ventricles are synchronous, and likewise those of the auricles; when the ventricles as in a state of disastole, the auricles are in a state of systole, and vice versa. The structure of the body of the heart is muscular, but about its base it is partly ligamentous or tendinous. The arteries originate in two trunks from the ventricles; the pulmonary artery emerges from the right ventricle, and ramifies through the lungs; the aorta arises from the left ventricle, and branches through every part of the body. Valves are stationed at the roots of the arteries, so as to hinder the return of the blood from arteries into the ventricles, without impeding the flow from the ventricles into the arteries. Arteries form cones, their apices at the heart, and their bases at their extreme capillaries. An artery is composed of several coats; but two only at present are worthy of our particular attention, namely, the muscular or irritable coat, and the elastic ... The coats of the veins possess both the irritable and elastic properties.[4]

Concept of Arterial Pulse

At the same time that Carson's above principles of cardiovascular functional anatomy were accepted in Britain, in France Bichat's widely read *Anatomie Générale* was available, having been published a few years earlier.[5] Bichat did not divide the circulation into general and pulmonary routes. He had devised the system of *red blood*, that commenced with the capillaries of the lungs, and the system of *black blood*, that began with the capillaries of the body. Thus, he had considered the sides of the heart as two distinct hearts, with each forming the intermediate organ between the veins and the arteries. Bichat proposed that fluids contained within the arteries were not absorbed, and that vital properties were extremely limited in the arterial system; the arterial tissue was destitute of cellular substance, and the circular fibers of the arteries were not muscular. Bichat taught, in correct distinction to many physiologists of the time, that the heart was the only power which gave motion to the blood, and that the vessels were purely passive, "obeying the motion which the heart communicated." He wisely stated that the limits of the heart's influence upon the blood were fixed within the capillary system, in which the fluid was transformed in color from red to black. Bichat's view of the pulse was also correct and contrary to many other medical leaders at the beginning of the nineteenth century. He proposed that

> the impulse of the blood is sudden and general, and derived from the heart; the locomotion of the arteries is the effect produced by this fluid, upon the walls of the vessels which transmit it. These together consitute the pulse. The first is essential to circulation. The second is not; and as it depends on the arterial structure, is subject to considerable varieties.[5]

Although Bichat did not believe that the arteries possessed irritability, i.e., the ability to respond to stimuli and contract (which we now know to be an important function, especially of small arterioles which can significantly control peripheral vascular resistance and capillary blood perfusion by smooth muscle contraction), he did make a speculation which has turned out to be gravely true. Bichat had stated, "fatal arrestations of circulation would be continually taking place if the arteries, like the intestines, possessed irritability."[5] We know now that of the group of interacting variables contributing to cerebral vascular, cardiovascular, and even intestinal vascular occulsions, which are often fatal, acute (spasm) and chronic (hypertension) pathophysiologic motor contraction of smooth muscle on the arterial side is an important element.

Bichat correctly believed that the arterial pulse depended only upon the systolic contraction of the heart, but others, such as Shearman,[6] believed that the arteries themselves rhythmically contracted, resulting in a detectible pulse. Dr. Parry, who agreed with Bichat, stated:

> The blood in every part of the arterial system may be considered as a set of continuous columns, possessing little compressibility, and filling the tubes in which they are contained. When, by the contraction of the left ventricle, the blood included in it is forcibly expelled into the aorta, all these columns receive the shock of propulsion at the same instant. But the velocity during this systole being greater than during the diastole, the momentum, and consequently the impulse, in every direction, is also greatest in the systole. When, therefore, an artery is compressed with the fingers, in the usual mode of feeling the pulse, the blood, in consequence of the systole rushing into the artery with an increase of momentum, gives a stronger impulse of dilation to the fingers, than from the less momentum which exists during the diastole, and thus produces the phenomenon of the pulse.[6]

Dr. William Shearman, in contrast to Bichat and Parry, interpreted the arterial pulse differently, suggesting,

> on the other hand, I would contend, that the pulsation is occasioned by an actual contraction of the vessel, restoring it to its former diameter previous to the reception of the additional quantity of blood thrown into the arteries during the systole of the heart.[6]

This view had earlier been ascribed to by Dumas, and even Galen, who maintained that the dilation and contraction of the arteries was an inherent property. Various arguments, both for and against arterial contraction, on normal and on physically denuded arteries, were presented between 1800 and 1825.[2]

Thus, the question of the nature and function of the arterial pulse was one of the chief topics of debate in early nineteenth century cardiovascular physiology.[7] In France, the renowned Magendie wrote on this topic in the *Journal de Physiologie Experimentale*.[8,9] Dr. Charles Bell, the respected surgeon in London, summarized the current quandary in 1819 when he stated[10]:

When we say that the blood returns or is returned (for we dare not be positive on this point) from the general venous system to the right auricle of the heart, from thence to the ventricle, from the ventricle to the lungs, from the lungs to the left side of the heart, and from thence to the general arterial system, we state almost the whole of our unquestioned knowledge relative to the circulation of this fluid. After all the experiments that have been made on the living and the dead — on the cold and the warm-blooded — with microscopes and with injections, the physiological world is as much divided on this interesting problem as in the days of Harvey. Independently of the numerous papers in periodical journals, four distinct works (Kerr, Carson, Parry, Bell) on the circulation of the blood have, within these two or three years, been published, and four *different* explanations attempted of what was supposed to be settled by Harvey. This is sufficient evidence that we have yet much to learn on the subject; and we think it behoves the different parties in this discussion to divert themselves, as much as possible, of preconceived opinions, and of that influence which great names impose, in order to be open to the arguments as well as the facts, brought forward by each other.

As stated earlier, Dr. Parry believed that arteries did not spontaneously contract or pulsate. Objections to his argument were that 1) It was contended that arteries must dilate and contract, because their dilatation was seen and felt, 2) That the pulse must arise from the dilatation and contraction, because this alternate movement was distinguishable by sight and touch, and 3) That arteries must, under common circumstances of circulation, dilate and contract *because* they were not "inert tubes," and because they had, under certain circumstances, an action independent of the heart. It is obvious that these objections to Dr. Parry's hypothesis, though held, were based upon a logical positivism which was at best, shallow. Dr. Charles Bell, supporting Parry's view that arterial pulsation was "occasioned by the whole quantity of blood sent through them in the direction of their axis," also stated that "Lewenhoek, the chief of microscopic observers, never saw the dilatation and contraction of arteries in the course of his multifarious experiments on the circulation of animals."[10] Bell also considered that because of

the alternate action of the diaphragm and abdominal muscles, the one receding while the other acts, that there is an uninterrupted pressure on the blood-vessels of this part of the body, and that respiration does not, therefore, accelerate the circulation of the blood in the abdomen.[11]

Earlier workers, such as Dumas and Galen believed that the dilatation and contraction of arteries were inherent in themselves, and independent of the mechanical impulse from the heart. Spalanzani concluded that arterial contractions were the cause of the pulse, though Spalanzani's experiments were "chiefly microscopical (the most fallacious of all experiments) and made on cold blooded-animals, as salamanders, lizards, frogs, etc."[2] Lucas contended in 1820 that "the fact of the pulse not being accompanied by any general dilatation of the arteries, in the ordinary state of the circulation, may, I hope, now be taken for granted...."[12] James Carson, who was Physician to the Workhouse, the Fever Hospital, and to the Asylum for the Pauper Lunatics, at Liverpool in 1815, did not believe arterial contraction to be necessary to propel blood,[13] but Charles Hastings of Edinburgh believed on the basis of dog, cat, and rabbit experiments, that it was.[14,15]

The notion of elasticity of the blood vessels was recognized early in the nineteenth century, and was considered as a factor in promoting circulation, as was muscular pulsatile contractions of blood vessels. Dr. Philip observed in 1823 that both the cardiac ventricles and arteries had elastic properties and that

> here, as in many other instances, both in men and the inferior animals, we see nature saving the muscular, by the substitution of the elastic power. The latter is the simplest, and its action tends little to exhaust it. In like manner the arteries are rendered elastic, to favour the ingress of the blood on the contraction of the ventricle. It is evident that a greater power must have been bestowed on the ventricle had the arteries been wholly inelastic. Their elasticity by resisting the pressure of the surrounding parts, and thus tending to preserve a uniformity of caliber, facilitates both the ingress and passage of the blood suddenly thrown into them. Had the blood entered by a continued stream, and been carried on merely by the power of the vessels themselves, this elasticity would not only have been of little use, but evidently injurious, as far as it tended to impede the muscular, or by whatever other name we choose to call that power by which the blood is propelled by the vessels. Thus it is that little elastic power is bestowed on the veins, which we shall find are unassisted in the propulsion of their contents.[16]

It was noted, for example by Dr. James Johnson in 1817,[17] that in some cases elasticity was lost in blood vessels of certain patients, as he observed upon autopsy that arteries were "totally converted into a bony tube," i.e. advanced atherosclerosis.

Dr. William Fennel of Virginia published his experiments and reflections[18] on elasticity and other properteries of arteries, in 1822. He assigned "two powers of motion to the animal machine — one its elasticity, the other its irritability."

> Elasticity appears to be a property given to parts, and only acts in subservience to the irritability: for instance, in an artery we have three states or capacities produced by three different causes, more particularly in the larger arteries. First, its dilated state — secondly, we have a contracted or diminished state — thirdly, its middle or pervious state. The first is dependent on the vis a tergo of the blood, derived from the systole of the heart — the second is dependent upon the contraction of the coats of the artery itself, produced by the stimulus of distention — the third is produced by the elasticity of the artery, and is independent of life.
> That the circulation may go on regularly, it is necessary that there should be some property inherent in the arteries, to keep them in that state which will favour the passage of the blood through them. No property could be better calculated to perform this office than elasticity, which confers on each

artery a tendency to remain pervious — or, in other words, keeps it open, that there may be as little retardment in the passage of the blood from the heart to the different parts of the body as possible.

As soon as the life or irritability of an artery is lost, its contractions cease — the elasticity becomes inactive, in as much as it has no power to withstand, and it necessarily must on this account rest in the middle state, or that state which shows the natural size of the part in possession of this property.

Now the chief office, as before observed, of the elasticity, appears to be that of keeping the arteries open, that they may receive the next gush of blood from the heart with as little impediment to its entrance as possible. I do not conceive that the elasticity of an artery can have the least influence in imparting velocity to the blood. It seems, indeed, to have an opposite effect, as the blood must overcome this power before the artery is dilated — and this power remaining the same, cannot throw the blood on with a greater force than was offered by the vis a tergo to overcome it.[18]

General Hydrostatics

Though concepts of the mechanisms of circulation were freely debated in the early nineteenth century, many writers firmly believed that whatever mechanisms existed, they were reducible to the fundamental laws of mathematics and the physics of hydrostatics. Examples of some of the known laws of hydrostatics, principles of the syphon, etc., are illustrated in the etchings reproduced in Fig. 23 and Fig. 24 from 1810.[19] Dr. Carson[13] conceived that the circulation of the blood could be reduced to the laws of hydrostatics. Dr. Young stated in 1809 that "the mechanical motions which take place in an animal body, are regulated by the same general laws as the motions of inanimate bodies" and

the motion of the blood is to be considered as that of a fluid, which obeys the laws of other fluids placed in the same circumstances; and, therefore the solution of the different problems respecting the progressive motion of the blood, as depending upon the muscular or elastic powers of the arteries, becomes a question in hydraulics, to be resolved by the acknowledged laws of this science, provided only that we are able distinctly to appreciate the nature of these powers.[20]

John Brickell, M.D., of Savannah, suggested in 1808[21] that there were "effects produced upon the circulation of the blood by its own gravity, (and that) the solution of this problem rested upon mathematical properties, which may be seen in the Principia of Sir Isaac Newton, Lib. 1, *de legibus motus*." Brickell diagramatically outlined the vector forces in relation to gravity and blood flow, and as well applied these concepts to certain disease states. Thus, relief of headache and ophthalmia might occur when placing the head to the zenith, leg pain and inflammation lessened by elevating the leg above the horizontal plane, etc.[21]

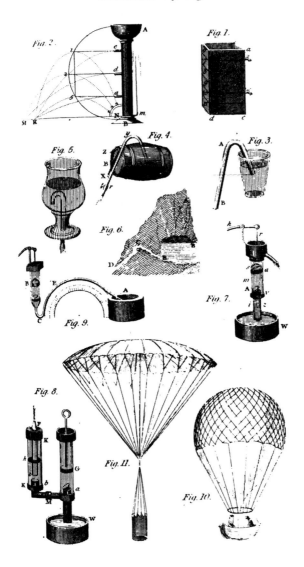

Fig. 23. Examples of hydrostatic principles, 1810. British etching (Joyce, 19).

James Alderson, a fellow of Pembroke College, Cambridge, applied similar concepts in describing motions of the heart in 1825.[22] He stated that

I am aware that mechanical physiologists are in no great repute at present, and probably no organ has contributed more to produce this opinion than the heart itself; still it must be admitted, that "with respect to mathematical reasoning in general, when it is cautiously applied, it has enabled us to arrive at physiological truths, which we perhaps could not have attained by

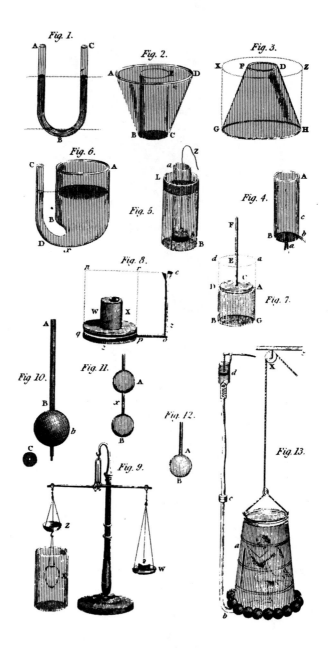

Fig. 24. Further examples of hydrostatic principles known in 1810. Taken from a British etching (Joyce, 19).

any other method, and which are beyond the reach of actual observation."* Alderson concluded that "the arch of the aorta may modify the heat's motion, ... but that the heart would have this motion independently of the aorta altogether, so long as the aortic orifice be out of the axis of the ventricle."[22]

Organ Circulation

It was recognized that the arterial system terminated in organ systems and glandular structures. Nicholl, in his outline of the circulation of the blood,[23] mentioned that arteries were supplied with nerves and were accompanied by nerves throughout their course, and sent terminating branches to glandular or secreting structures. After injection of coloring materials, such as the blue prussiate of potash, Dr. Mayer, professor of anatomy at Berne, observed the transport of this dye to many organs in the body, including the salivary glands, pancreas, and mammillary glands, but not the bones or bone marrow. He also administered this agent to a pregnant animal and demonstrated

> the fact of a direct passage of fluids from the mother to the foetus; a fact which physiology had hitherto in vain endeavoured to ascertain. Fluids passing into the blood of the mother are deposited in the cellular tissue of the placenta, and are absorbed by the veins of the foetus.[24]

Studies on the "absorbing powers of the veins and lymphatics" were published by Lawrence and Coates in 1823,[25] and Home also discussed the relative importance of the thoracic duct in carrying fluids from the stomach to the circulating blood.[26] After placing the blue prussiate directly into the intestine of the experimental animal, the former investigators concluded that most of it was transported by the thoracic duct. Their data are illustrated in Table 4.[25] (See also the chapter on Gastrointestinal Function for further details on gut circulation.)

The circulation to the lungs was discussed by Harlan in 1819, and, on the basis of experiments with cats, Harlan concluded that the circulation of blood through the lungs was "immediately and entirely suppressed during expiration."[27] He also made reasonable (at least in part) recommendations for resuscitation after asphyxia, including

> 1) Mechanical inflation of the lungs, 2) To restore the temperature of the body by the warm bath, friction, etc., 3) Stimuli, external and internal; as enemata of brandy, etc., and 4) To evacuate the contents of the stomach.

A detailed explanation of circulation to the head was published by Dr. James Carson of Liverpool, in 1824.[4] His anatomic description was quite ac-

---

Bostock, Elementary Treatise on Physiology, *Vol. i, p. 416, as re-quoted by James Alderson.*[22]

Table 4
Experimental Data (1823) of Lawrence and Coates
Showing Distribution of Blue Prussiate of Potash in Various
Circulatory Routes After Intra-intestinal Administration[25]

Animals	Quantity	Thoracic Duct	Carotid and Jugular	Urine
Kitten	½ oz. of solution	12 and 13 m.* distinct blue	6 m. distinct blue	19 m. no blue
Idem	Idem	4 m. blue	2 m. no blue	10 or 15 m. no blue 29 m. distinct blue
Idem	Idem nearly	3¾ m. blue	2 m. no blue	5 m. blue, not strongly
Idem	½ oz.	3 m. blue	4 m. strongly blue	More than 4 m. doubtful
Cat	Uncertain	9½ m. blue	6 m. no blue	More than 9½ m. no blue

*m = minutes after injection

curate and complete, as the state of gross anatomy was much more advanced than physiology in the early nineteenth century. The peculiar nature of cranial circulation, with the presence of ventricles and sinuses in the brain and the less variable circulation of this organ, compared to other organs, with changes in physiologic status were noted by Carson. He observed that

> the arteries, which convey the blood to the head, throw this fluid into the cranium by synchronous jets. An equal quantity, according to the hypothesis contended for, must at the same instant be discharged from the cranium into the veins. This must also be by jets, which cause successive currents, or, in other words, pulsations in these veins. While the contents of the ventricles, and the substance of the brain, remain unaltered, it is evident, that the quantity of blood contained in the cranium must be at all times the same. No force could, in the state supposed, increase this quantity of blood; and from this circumstance, a great security is given to the vessels of the brain, the rupture of any of which would be attended with fatal effects. Nor would the abstraction of any quantity of blood from the rest of the system, diminish that contained within the cranium.[4]

Dr. Carson also summarized important conclusions, made earlier by Dr. Monro (Fig. 25), on the cerebrospinal fluid of the ventricles, and of hydrocephalus. He stated:

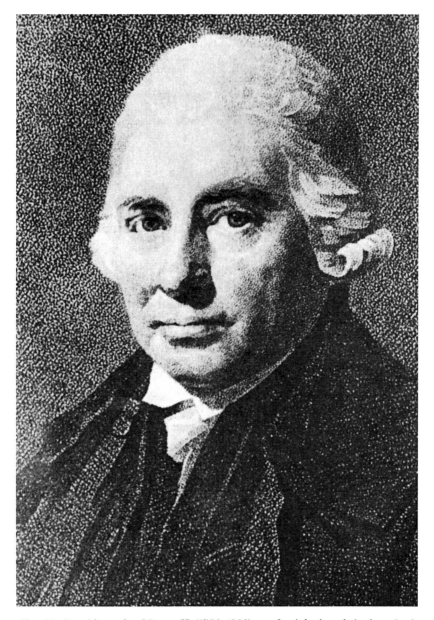

Fig. 25. Dr. Alexander Monro II (1756–1823), a physiologist of the lymphatic system (painted by Sir Henry Raeburn).

Previously to the time of Dr. Monro, and by many physicians of the present day, in the case of accumulation of water in the ventricles, the water was supposed to compress the brain into smaller bulk. Dr. Monro justly contended against this opinion, and maintained, that the water, in these circumstances, by pressing against the brain, caused the absorption of that organ; and that, by this means, a part of this substance of the brain was consumed, or rather dislodged from the encephalon, to give room for this increased quantity of water. An opinion was held by Dr. Monro, and indeed by all the physiologists of his day, that the office of absorption was solely performed by a peculiar class of vessels called lymphatics. Though the search had occupied the eager and ambitious toil of anatomists during the last fifty years of the 18th century, no lymphatic vessels could ever be found in the brain. It was concluded from this, that water, when once deposited in the ventricles, or in any part of the encephalon, must remain there, as there existed no machinery by which it could be removed. In the case of the disease called *hydrocephalus*, Dr. Monro was induced to recommend as the only, but awful alternative, the discharging of the water by puncture of the brain.[4]

Microscopic Analyses of Circulation

Blood capillary function was discussed at length by several writers, including the French physician, Sarlandiere[28] and Bichat in his *Anatomie Générale*.[5] Bichat concluded that "the blood of the capillaries is beyond the influence of the heart; hence the frequently opposite periods of action in the heart and capillaries ..." though he was of course wrong in this interpretation. Spallanzani undertook microscopic studies of capillary circulation in 1771–1802, using the

> anatomical instrument of Lyonet, which is an improvement upon that of Lewenhoek. He long doubted whether the reasoning founded upon phenomena observed in the circulation of cold blooded animals, would apply to the warm; but at last, in May 1771, he observed distinctly by the microscope, in an incubated egg, the circulation of the blood in the arteries and veins.[29]

Dr. Wilson Philip also used the microscope to study microcirculation in 1816. He reported:

> I have found, by the assistance of the microscope, both in warm and cold blooded animals, that the motion of the blood in the smaller vessels continues for a very long time after what we call death, although immediately after it a ligature be thrown round all the vessels attached to the heart, and this organ be removed. I have seen it continue in the mesentery of a rabbit, for more than an hour after the removal of the heart, even where the bowels had been hanging out of the abdomen for the whole of this time, and had become dry and cold.[30]

This same investigator also investigated the frog, whose heart had been extirpated, and stated,

> on bringing the web of one of the hind legs before the microscope, I found

the circulation in it vigorous, I could not distinguish it from that in the web of a healthy frog. It continued in this state for many minutes, and, at length, gradually became more languid.[16]

Dr. Philip also examined the intestinal mesentery of the rabbit by microscopy, and concluded

that the motion of the blood in the capillaries, that is, those vessels which are too small to be distinguished by the naked eye, has no direct dependence on the action of the heart. Does it depend on a power remaining in the larger vessels, or on the power of the capillaries themselves? This point also may easily be determined by direct experiment. If it depends on the former, it will be influenced by stimulants and sedatives acting on the capillaries; if on the latter, the velocity of the blood will be greater or less according as they are more or less excited. I found from many experiments ... that the velocity of the blood in the capillaries is immediately influenced by the state of these vessels. When they were stimulated by the concentrated rays of the sun, the application of spirits of wine, or gentle friction, the velocity of the blood in them was immediately, and, by the two first, to a great degree increased. When the power of the capillaries was destroyed, even in the perfect animal, by the direct application of an infusion of opium or tobacco to them, the motion of the blood through them immediately ceased.[16]

The early microscope was also used, by Mr. Howship, to study the microcirculation of bone and cartilage. Howship concluded

that, in the mammalia, the first rudiments of ossification in the long bones are the effect of a secreting power in the arteries, upon the internal surface of the periosteum, which produce a portion of a hollow cylinder; this form of bone having been found antecedent to the evolution of any cartilaginous structure ...

and

that while the circulation in the capillary arteries situated between the cartilage and bone must provide the phosphate of lime, the principal agent in extending the cylinder, and in effecting the subsequent progressive changes of structure, which in a growing bone are continually taking place, appears to be simply the mechanical pressure exerted by the fluid secretions within the medullary cavities of bone, this power operating successively in different directions, according to the particular determination given by the circulation.[31]

Circulatory Disorders

Diseases of the cardiovascular system were very poorly understood during the dawn of the nineteenth century. Chronic diseases of cardiovascular origin, so common today in elderly patients, were significantly less common in that period when most mortality and morbidity was due to infectious and other diseases. Hypertension, when it did occur was not measurable at that time; even today it is often undiagnosed because it is frequently nonsymptomatic. Arteriosclerosis was not understood, nor was the basis of peripheral vascular disease. Only those entities associated with obvious anatomic defects, seen upon gross dissection after death, were identifiable, such as arterial aneurysms, infectious abscesses localized to the heart, or other gross degenerative states. The English surgeon, Joseph Hodgson (1788-1868), published *A Treatise on the Diseases of Arteries and Veins* in 1815.[32] Classical descriptions of aortic aneurysms were published by Hodgson in this book, and the gifted medical artist, Antonio Scarpa[39] prepared outstanding engravings of aortic aneurysms, the innervation of the heart (Fig. 26), and other cardiovascular subjects. Scarpa also suggested that arterial walls might become degenerate due to syphilis, and Dr. Baldwin of the new United States of America described left ventricular abscesses of unknown origin.[33] Aortic aneurysms were also described in France by Bourdon[34] and in Scotland Nicoll published a case history of aneurysm of the femoral arteries of a bricklayer. The latter case was treated surgically, with recovery of the patient.[35]

Few advances were made clarifying the nature of cardiovascular diseases in France during the period 1800–1825, in large part due to the erroneous conceptions of the relationship between inflammation, circulation and disease.[36] Broussais and his disciple, Vialle, advanced their theory on "inequilibrium in the balance of the circulation and excitability, as the principal source and phenomenon in most diseases."[37] Broussais taught that "it is principally to inflammation in the mucous membranes — more rarely in the serous tissues or parenchymatous structures of the internal viscera, we owe those various fevers, hitherto denominated *idiopathic*." Broussais' teachings in France were translated into English but British editors did not support his concepts, saying

> We have preferred giving this detailed view (English Translation) of a most important doctrine, to the collection of a heterogeneous mass of curiosities of monstrosities, which would never bear a second reading. We venture to predict that ... (his teachings) will not only produce a considerable sensation in the medical world here, but have a salutary influence on the treatment of disease when the spirit that conceived, and the hand that transcribed it shall have fled to the skies or mouldered in the tomb![37]

Technical Advances in Cardiology

As a result of an environment which encouraged experimental inquiry during the early nineteenth century, several significant technological procedures were developed and an enhanced factual understanding of cardiology resulted during this era. These advances covered such things as cardiac auscultation, improved descriptive atlases on cardiac diseases, blood transfusion, intravenous administration of foreign agents, etc. Each one of these was

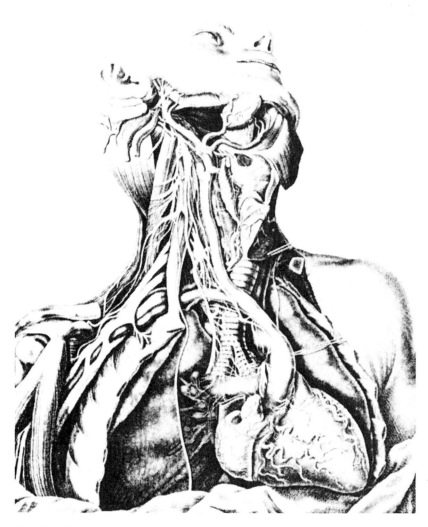

Fig. 26. The nerves of the heart, drawn by Antonio Scarpa (1747-1832). Taken from Plate III of Scarpa's "Tabulae Nevrologicae ad Illustrandam Historiam Anat. Cardiacorum Nervorum," etc., 1794. This was the first accurate delineation of the nerves of the heart.

not entirely novel to the time period, 1800–1825, but each was an important field for development.

In the early nineteenth century methods of clinical examination were still very primitive. Percussion for sounding the thorax had been employed since the time of Hipprocrates, and cardiac auscultation by the direct method of placing the physician's ear on the patient's chest had been described since the twelfth century. René Theophil Hyacinthe Laennec of France is credited with developing the first stethoscope for cardiac auscultation. He had been frustrated with auscultation by the direct method, claiming it

> as uncomfortable for the doctor as it was for the patient, (thus) ... making it impracticable in hospitals. It was hardly suitable where most women were concerned, and with some the size of their breasts was a physical obstacle to the employment of the method for examination of the heart and lungs.[38]

In 1806, Laennec's initial development of a stethoscope began on his way to visit a stout young lady with heart disease. He observed some boys playing in the courtyard of the Louvre, one of which held a long wooden beam to his ear while another boy struck the other end, and transmitted the sound in this manner. Laennec therefore was able to transfer this concept to the hearing of heart sounds, and undertook early experiments with a large variety of instruments made from rolled paper, ebony, malacca cane, cedar, lime wood, glass and metal. Eventually he settled upon a thick-walled tube about a foot long, made of beech wood, for auscultation of breath sounds and rales, and adapted with a stopper in the funnel for detecting heart sounds. This instrument, reported by Laennec in 1818, became known as the pectoriloquy or medical trumpet. Others in this era also became expert in the medical use of the stethoscope, including James Hope (1801–1841), a medical student in Edinburgh, who used the stethoscope for his 1825 M.D. thesis on aneurysm of the aorta. Hope later became a famous cardiologist, and published *Diseases of the Heart* in 1831, which was the best book on this subject at the time.[39] Jacques Alexandre Le Jumeau Kergaradec was one of the first (others have been credited with this distinction including Mayor of Geneva in 1818 and Phillipe Le Goust in 1650) to hear fetal heart sounds. He was a friend and contemporary of Laennec, and used the Laennec stethoscope to study fetal heart sounds.

Another technical advance in cardiology was by Antonio Scarpa (1747?–1832). Scarpa was a student and assistant of the aged and famous Morgagni, and became appointed Professor of Anatomy and Clinical Surgery at Modena, Italy, in 1772. He also studied in Vienna, London, and Paris and reported on aortic aneurysm at the French Royal Society of Medicine. Becoming something of an expert on aneurysms, he published a treatise on this subject in 1804, as well as an earlier outstanding atlas, *Tabulae Nevrologicae ad Illustrandam Historiam Anat. Cardiocorum Nervorum, etc.* in 1794.[39] In 1815 knowledge of aneurysms was further enhanced by publication of another major work, *A Treatise on the Diseases of Arteries and Veins* by the English surgeon, Joseph Hodgson.[40]

Dr. E. Hale, of Boston, reported in 1821 his experiments with intravenous injection, including his experiments with rabbits and with himself as an experimental subject.[41] His report was one of the very few original papers on intravenous administration to humans, inasmuch as he mentioned a single earlier report by Fabricius and Smith which he had not himself read. Before

Hale's investigation many workers had attempted intravenous injections only on animals, and his 1821 report with rabbits showed that intravenous administration of colocynth, ipecacuanha, rhubarb, tarter emetic, etc., at the doses he used, were relatively nontoxic. His rabbit experiments with intravenous administration of sulphate of magnesia, calcined magnesia, or alcohol resulted in rapid death of the animals. Hale's philosophic rationalization for animal versus human experimentation is worth repeating:

> Much may be presumed, much fairly inferred with regard to the human subject from what happens in experiments made upon animals; and all new experiments judiciously performed may serve to strengthen and confirm the deductions which have already been made—but although an approach is thus constantly made to certainy in our conclusions—that certainty is never reached; as in a circulating decimal every recurrence of the repetend brings it nearer to an unit, and yet if infinitely repeated it never arrives at it. Every instance in which a medicinal substance is injected into the veins of an animal, and an effect is produced which corresponds to the known qualities of that substance, and this too without any injurious consequences to the life or health of the animal employed from the operation itself, renders it more and more probable that the practice might be extended with safety and propriety to individuals of our own species—and yet no number of such instances would perfectly satisfy us that the practice was advisable, or would be successful till the attempt had actually been made.[41]

Dr. Hale undertook his experimental intravenous injection upon himself on February 20, 1820, and followed up on his physiologic responses for four weeks. His account, in which he administered castor oil, began as follows:

> Having been persuaded, from my own observation, and those of others, that some of the milder medicines may be injected into the veins with safety, I resolved to make the experiment upon myself. Accordingly I filled a half ounce measure with cold pressed castor oil, and placed it in a basin of water of the temperature of 100°; one drachm of it, I drew into a syringe, and placed this also in the basin; it being my intention first to inject one drachm ... When I had made all the preparations which I thought necessary, I sat down and counted my pulse, and found it to beat eighty times a minute ... An assistant (a medical student) placed a ligature round my left arm, as in the common operation for bleeding, and opened the median vein by a pretty large orifice ... He then attempted to introduce the silver tube, while I held a bowl to receive the blood, which flowed very freely. But being a little agitated, he was not able to get the tube into the orifice in the vein. As there was no time to be lost, I took the tube myself, and after several ineffectual trials, which gave considerable pain, I succeeded in introducing it. We immediately took off the ligature and began to inject the oil. The hemorrhage ceased as soon as the ligature was loosened; we estimated that about eight ounces of blood was lost, before that was done.

Dr. Hale continued his description, hour by hour, of his responses which, fortunately, only elicited moderate problems of catharsis, nausea, taste of castor oil, dizziness, and several days later, general weakness, stiffness of the injected arm, a hematoma, etc. His final conclusion was

> Let the circumstances be what they may under which the operation is performed, let the care taken be ever so great, let the operator be ever so skilful, we apprehend that in the human subject the injection of any medicinal substance, especially any one of sufficient power to make its introduction an object, could never be an operation free from hazard, and danger to life.[41]

Today intravenous injections of medicinal agents, fluid and salt replacement materials, and dietary substances are routine, yet we know that materials injected and instrumentation used must be sterile, that toxic dose levels are rapidly and dangerously reached, and that air bubbles must not be injected. Therefore, Hale's pioneering work with himself was hazardous for reasons beyond his own realization, he was lucky that his response was not fatal, and his observed adverse responses most probably resulted from an injection from contaminated castor oil or dirty equipment used. Nonetheless, his report and wilingness for self-sacrifice helped advance medicine.

The transfusion of blood was not a novel concept originating in the early nineteenth century, though it was seldom undertaken on humans in this era. Both the alleged superabundance of blood, which was the theoretical basis for blood-letting, and the harmful effects of hemorrhage were discussed prior to 1825, but blood transfusion experiments were usually performed on animals. The earliest human blood transfusion was accredited to Francis Folli in 1654, though this case is not well documented. In 1665, Dr. Richard Lower of Cornwall successfully transfused blood from one animal to another.[42] By 1824 the English physiologist and obstetrician, James Blundell, made the first transfusion of human blood into a human patient. In his reports, he concluded that blood from animals of one species was not suitable for that of another species, and that venous blood was as satisfactory as arterial blood. Others, such as Leacock[43] stated in 1817 that

> it appears clear, from a candid review of [his] ... experiments, that the blood of any animal, transfused into the vascular system of another animal of the same species, is sufficient to support life ... It is not, however, quite clear, that animals of *different species* will bear this transfusion to a great extent. For example, ... [his one] experiment shows that the blood of a sheep, an herbivorous animal, may support a dog, a carnivorous animal.

Leacock further stated that "I bled a cat from the jugular vein till syncope ensued. I then transfused the blood of a dog I had in readiness, in a very small stream, into the vein of a cat. She soon revived, and afterwards recovered."[43] Other cross-species transfusions of Leacock failed, with fatal results. As shown in Figure 27, with its descriptive commentary, Leacock designed a practical blood transfusion tube from an ox's ureter and crow quills.

I made a small incision for receiving a pipe between the middle ligature and hat farthest from the heart, which had been drawn tight. Keeping in readiness the upper ligature to stop hæmorrhage, I opened a communication between the two dogs thus :

I took a tube [*a a a*] about six inches long, made of an ox's ureter, and secured to each end of it a crow-quill; [*β b*] one of which [*β*] I introduced into the quill [*c*] which was attached to the jugular vein of the small dog; while that which was secured to the artery of the other animal [*d*] was introduced into the quill of the tube [*b*]. Every thing being now ready, I removed the forceps from the femoral artery of the large dog, when the blood passed rapidly into the vein of the other, through the artificial channel. In two minutes, the receiving dog that had been lying half dead, raised his head ; the pulse, before imperceptible, began to be plainly felt ; the eye that was previously dull and glassy, regained its former splendour; the respiration became easy and natural. — Soon afterwards he became impatient, and attempted to escape. I now put an end to the experiment : the dog ran about with ease, and appeared very little indisposed.

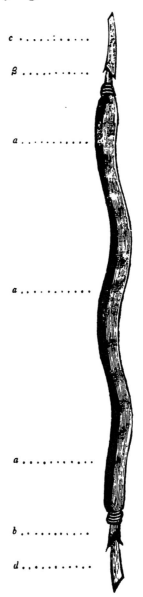

Fig. 27. Dr. Leacock's transfusion tube, constructed from an ox ureter and crow quills, in 1817.

In view of modern knowledge of the high specificity of blood types, even within one species, it is remarkable that a higher percentage of fatal and delayed adverse reactions was not reported after inter-species and intra-species experimental transfusions.

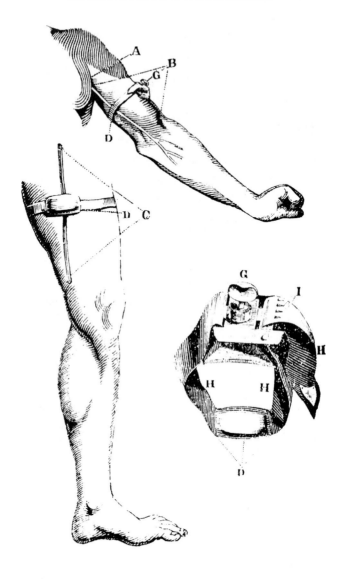

Fig. 28. Etching showing the design of an early nineteenth century tourniquet (Great Britain).

Enlightenment about some of the physical properties of blood aided in the transfusion of blood. Defibrinated blood was found to be as suitable as whole blood for transfusion, and Prevost and Dumas (1821) were able to prevent blood coagulation by means of adding an anticoagulant to the whole blood.[42] Detailed etchings for the design of a proper tourniquet were also published in this period (Figure 28).

The Formation, Color, and Coagulation of Blood

Ideas on the formation of blood were understandably vague and incorrect in the early nineteenth century. One commonly held view was that all the food and drink consumed was directly converted to blood, via absorption in the intestines into the thoracic duct (which we now know contains white or clear lymph with a pinkish hue), whereupon it later emptied into the main vascular system.[44]

Chemical analyses of blood serum were reported to the Society for the Improvement of Animal Chemistry in 1812 by William Brande.[45] He concluded that serum contained "gelatine, uncombined soda, minute portions of saline substances, such as muriate of soda and potash, and phosphate of lime, ammonia, and slight traces of oxide of iron." The "electric phenomena" of blood were described by Dr. Bellingeri in 1824.[46] This Italian medical specialist attested that during cases of severe inflammation, blood was negatively electrified, but in normal health held only a small degree of electricity. The red color of blood was of debatable origin during the early nineteenth century, but many "respectable physiologists" believed it to be due to the red oxide of iron in blood.[47,48] By 1800 the anatomists had divided the components of blood into serum, red globules, and coagulating lymph. In addition to the gelatin and chemicals of blood described above by Brande, fiber was considered an important constituent of the "clot of crassamentum." According to James Parkinson of London (1801), "This substance (fibrin) may be regarded as that part of the blood which has undergone the most complete animalization; and from which the muscular fibre and other organs of the body are formed."[49] The above conclusion on blood color and fibrin composition, formulated around 1800 when the chemistry of proteins and oxyhemoglobin were not yet unravelled, were remarkably sound. Though muscle and other organ proteins are not formed from fibrin, there is a similar macromolecular structure of the proteins constituting muscle and blood fibrin which imparts a similar gross, physical property. Further, the red color of blood is due to the red color of heme, especially in its oxygenated state, contained in blood corpuscles, and which is in fact attributable to the iron contained in the hemoglobin molecule.

The coagulation of blood was subject to considerable experimentation in the early nineteenth century in attempts to discover the mechanism of this phenomenon. Dr. Thomas Hewson was one investigator in this field. He considered the possible roles of heat, agitation, exposure to air, etc., as important factors in the coagulation of blood. His following account,[50] published in 1811, was the basis of his conclusion that *air* was the "strong coagulant of the blood," and not cold nor rest (absence of circulation).

> As the temperature of the human body generally surpasses that of the circumambient air, it has been inferred, that the coagulation of the blood, like the congelation of water, depended on the mere abstraction of heat. The analogy of size, and animal jelly, which are fluid in the temperature of our

bodies, and become solid when exposed to the medium temperature of the atmosphere, seems to give strength to this opinion. There is, however, this essential difference, that water and jelly assume the solid or fluid state, according to the degree of heat which is applied (but when once blood has coagulated, it is incapable of being rendered fluid by any additional heat. And farther, it has been very satisfactorily proved by the experiments of Mr. Hewson and Mr. Hunter, that the blood may be actually frozen and converted into ice before it has time to coagulate; and yet on being thawed it coagulates like blood that had never been frozen. Mr. Hewson has likewise shown that the blood coagulates as readily when placed in a heat of 100°, which is equal to the natural temperature of our bodies, as in a heat of 67°, and a heat of 120° produces a more immediate coagulation.

The continual agitation which the blood undergoes during its circulation through the body, has been considered by many as the principal means of maintaining its fluidity; and it has been urged, that rest alone was sufficient to occasion the coagulation of the blood. In support of this opinion, its advocates have adduced the familiar experiment of agitating the blood, when received in a basin, by means of a bunch of rods or small sticks; in which case it is asserted the coagulation will be prevented. If we scrutinize into the circumstances attendant on this experiment, there will be no difficulty in detecting the nature of the deception, and in showing the complete futility of the argument. In fact, the coagulation is complete, and the sticks will be found loaded with solid matter, that part of the blood which is alone capable of spontaneous coagulation, and freed from it, the other parts remain in their natural fluid state.

With the view of acquiring more precise ideas respecting the comparative influence of agitation or rest in the coagulation of the blood, I made the following experiments. About six ounces of blood were received, from a vein in the arm, in a white earthen bowl; the time required for collecting this quantity was three minutes. While the blood was yet flowing from the vein, it was kept constantly agitated with a small bunch of slender sticks. In five minutes the coagulation had evidently commenced, and at the end of five minutes more it appeared to be complete. The whole time occupied in this experiment was thirteen minutes. After the removal of the small clot which adhered to the sticks, the remaining blood was set apart for further examination; and on the next day it still continued fluid, a proof that the whole of the coagulating principle had been removed. In farther confirmation it may be mentioned, that the coagulum, when washed and dried, weighed thirteen grains, equal to the largest proportion of fibrine, I have ever been able to detect in the blood.

Immediately as the first bowl was removed a similar one was employed to receive a like quantity of blood; and here the time occupied in collecting it was likewise three minutes. It was not till the end of ten minutes after it was set by the rest, that there was any appearance of coagulation, and five minutes more were required before it was complete, making in all a period of eighteen minutes.[50]

In France at the famous hospital, Hotel Dieu, Dr. M. Belhomme published over five hundred experiments made on blood, many with respect to its coagulation.[51] The formation of the "buffy coat" upon the coagulum was considered noteworthy, and comparisons in clotting times of blood withdrawn from diseased versus healthy subjects were made. Belhomme observed a constant tendency for the blood of pregnant women to exhibit a buffy coat. He further distinguished "that the blood of females in this state yields a smell decidedly like that of a placenta recently thrown off — a phenomenon always observed by him; and which, in doubtful cases of pregnancy, may be of the greatest importance." This test for pregnancy appeared not to be adopted by his fellow physicians.

Chapter V

Smallpox Vaccination: A Successful Community Approach

Smallpox, a virally-induced and usually fatal disease, was one of the leading contributors to mortality in Europe and the New World in the 18th and 19th centuries. Until its virtual and very recent eradication worldwide in the 1970's, it had remained the dreaded killer of thousands of inhabitants of South America, Africa, India and China even through the 1960's. The principles employed for its ultimate defeat during current times were those developed and exploited on a community-wide scale for the first time in the early nineteenth century.

Early History

The time and exact location for the earliest origin of smallpox are lost in antiquity and debated by historical scholars, and perhaps occurred in ancient Rome or Greece, but it is accepted that the first recognizable account of smallpox was written by the Chinese scholar, Ko Hung, who lived from 265–313 A.D. Evidence of smallpox occurred, amongst other times, in Europe in 581 A.D. and 980 A.D., but it became much more common and more lethal in the 18th and 19th centuries. The repeated exposures to smallpox and the existence of a mild form, *Variola minor* (alastrim), imparted a weak resistance to the more virulent form, *Variola major* in European inhabitants, a phenomenon not demonstrated in New World natives when European explorers sailed to Mexico and the West Indies, bringing smallpox to the New World. Thus, during the period 1519–1548 when Cortez and other Conquistadores visited Mexico, smallpox contributed greatly to the destruction of the Aztec race. Epidemics were recorded in 1520, 1531, 1545, 1564, 1576, and 1595 in Mexico, and 18.5 million of a total population of 25 million were decimated by this disease in New Spain.[1] In Europe the character of the smallpox pestilence began to change in the eighteenth century, and it became more virulent and more selectively attacked children. Eighty percent of smallpox deaths in London, 1769–1774, were in children under five and during this era smallpox was

Table 5
Proportion of Smallpox Mortality
to Total Mortality (1804–1818)
in London, as Reported by Sir Gilbert Blane[3]

Years	Total Mortality	Mortality from Small Pox	Proportion		Proportion to 1000
1804	17,038	622	1 in 27½		36
1805	17,565	1685	1	10	96
1806	18,334	1297	1	14	71
1807	17,938	1158	1	15½	65
1808	19,964	1169	1	17¼	58
1809	16,680	1163	1	14¼	70
1810	19,893	1198	1	16½	60
1811	17,043	751	1	22¾	44
1812	18,295	1287	1	14¼	70
1813	17,322	898	1	19¼	52
1814	19,783	638	1	31	32
1815	19,560	725	1	27	37
1816	20,316	653	1	31¼	32
1817	19,968	1051	1	19	53
1818	19,705	421	1	47	21
Total	279,404	14,716	1 in 18.9		53

endemic in Europe causing thousands of deaths per year, with periodic flare-ups of great epidemics. Later the disease was to become less prevalent in small villages and in the very young, and would exert its toll mostly within the larger cities and slums. In London alone, from 1723 until the turn of the century, sizable outbreaks of smallpox occurred at intervals ranging from 2 to 11 years, with over 3,000 deaths in each outbreak. At the same time nearly 19 percent of all deaths in Glasgow were attributable to smallpox.[2] Table 5, which is taken directly from Sir Gilbert Blane's 1819 "Statement of Facts Tending to Establish an Estimate of the True Value and Present State of Vaccination," and published in the *Medico-Chirurgical Transactions*,[2] illustrates data from the mortality bills in London indicating the high mortality from smallpox. In the preceding 15 year period, before vaccination was used in London, the mortality rate was almost double that shown in Table 5.

Man is the only reservoir of the smallpox virus, which is an organism transmitted through the air, probably in water droplets, from patients with the active disease; carriers without the active disease do not exist. Accordingly, smallpox is an acutely acquired disease and the patient is infectious from the prodromal period through the time in which the skin lesions or their crusts exist. The lesions, which cover the entire body, are the hallmark of this disease, and these areola pass through stages of pustulation and subsequently crust formation, eventually leaving scars or pock marks, if the patient survives.

The contageousness of smallpox was naturally recognized in its early history, but in this premicrobiologic period the mode of transmission was unknown. Medical literature in the early nineteenth century referred to a "virus" as a causative agent, but this was a general term applied to unknown agents of contagion, and the modern use of this word in reference to specific types of replicating, microbiologic organisms did not apply in the early 1800's. Immunity to smallpox was noted, and it was early established that patients who recovered from an affliction of smallpox did not become afflicted a second time, even if exposed to patients with the active disease. Attempts to create immunity to smallpox by various means, including inoculation and vaccination, were made, and the development of vaccination during the early nineteenth century indeed constituted one of the milestones in the advancement of preventative medicine. The widespread use of vaccination, resulting from the early clinical experimentation and technical development by Edward Jenner, was one of the first attempts to combat disease at the national level, in several countries, and to protect communities rather than only the individual.

The principle of inoculation did not begin with Jenner, but had existed for over 800 years prior to his time inasmuch as it was practiced by Chinese physicians in the eleventh century and before that in India. Chinese physicians ground the dried crusts of smallpox vesicles and blew the powder into the nose of their patients in attempts to confer immunity. One of the earliest European accounts of inoculation against smallpox, in the 18th century, was that of Giacomo Pylarini of Smyrna, Greece, who transferred the liquid from smallpox pustules to scratch marks on the recipient to protect the individual. Inoculation by this manner became popular during the early 18th century, but was accompanied by an estimated 2–3 percent mortality induced by the inoculation procedure (the ensuing attack not always being mild), and furthermore, inoculation by fresh smallpox material tended to spread the incidence of this contagious disease to multiple points in the community. Thus, in Europe, where the population density was higher than in the developing United States, smallpox inoculation became disfavored by 1728 due to these problems. The attacks of smallpox induced by inoculation, which were usually mild, could however be more easily isolated in the less densely settled America, and the practice of inoculation persisted in the new United States throughout the eighteenth century.

Dr. Jenner's Report

The principle of vaccination consists, in short, of inoculating into humans or animals a virus of one type, which by itself will produce only a mild reaction, but which will induce in the host immunity to a virus of more dangerous character. Thus, antibodies induced in humans during the immune response to the cowpox virus, will confer immunity to the similar, but more harmful smallpox virus. Accidental observations of this phenomenon with respect to cowpox were observed prior to Dr. Edward Jenner's work, but Dr. Jenner (Fig. 29) was the initial developer and reporter of the serendipitous finding. His own words describing this observation, published in 1801[4] were as follows:

> My inquiry into the nature of the Cow-pox commenced upwards of twenty-five years ago. My attention to this singular disease was first excited by observing, that among those whom in the country I was frequently called upon to inoculate, many resisted every effort to give them the Small-pox. These patients I found had undergone a disease they called the Cow-pox, contracted by milking cows affected with a peculiar eruption on their teats. On inquiry, it appeared that it had been known among the dairies since time immemorial, and that a vague opinion prevailed that it was a preventive of the Small-pox. This opinion I found was, comparatively, new among them; for all the older farmers declared they had no such idea in their early days—a circumstance that seemed easily to be accounted for, from my knowing that the common people were very rarely inoculated for the Small-pox, till that practice was rendered general by the improved method introduced by the Suttons: so that the working people in the dairies were seldom put to the test of the preventive powers of the Cow-pox.
>
> In the course of the investigation of this subject, which, like all others of a complex and intricate nature, presented many difficulties, I found that some of those *who seemed to have undergone the Cow-pox*, nevertheless, on inoculation with the Small-pox, felt its influence just the same as if no disease had been communicated to them from the cow. This occurrence led me to enquire among the medical practitioners, in the country around me, who all agreed in this sentiment, that the Cow-pox was not to be relied upon as a certain preventive of the Small-pox. This for a while damped but did not extinguish my ardour; for as I proceeded, I had the satisfaction to learn that the cow was subject to some varieties of spontaneous eruptions upon her teats; that they were all capable of communicating sores to the hands of the milkers; and that whatever sore was derived from the animal, was called in the dairy the Cow-pox. Thus, I surmounted a great obstacle, and, in consequence, was led to form a distinction between these diseases, one of which only I have denominated the *true*, the others the *spurious*, Cow-pox, as they possess no specific power over the constitution. This impediment to my progress was not long removed, before another, of far greater magnitude in its appearances, started up. There were not wanting instances to prove, that when the true Cow-pox broke out among the cattle at a dairy, a person who had milked an infected animal, and had thereby apparently gone through the disease in common with others, was liable to receive the Small-pox afterwards. This, like the former obstacle, gave a painful check to my fond and aspiring hopes: but reflecting that the operations of Nature are generally uniform, and that it was not probable the human constitution (having undergone the Cow-pox) should in some instances be perfectly shielded from the Small-pox, and in many others remain unprotected, I resumed my labours with redoubled ardour. The result was fortunate; for I now discovered that the virus of Cow-pox was liable to undergo progressive changes, from the same causes precisely as that of Small-pox; and that when it was applied to the Human skin in its degenerated state, it would produce the ulcerative effects in as great a degree as when it was not decomposed, and sometimes far greater; but having lost *its specific proper-*

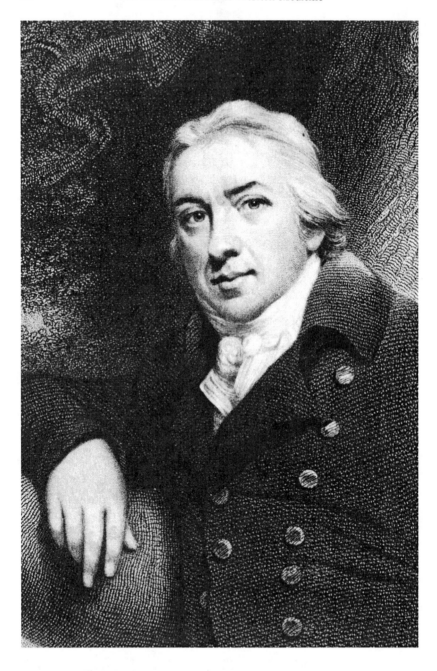

Fig. 29. Dr. Edward Jenner (1749–1823). Based upon earlier concepts of inoculation against smallpox, Jenner transformed a local country tradition, vaccination, into a successful prophylactic procedure with widespread public health benefits.

Table 6

Number of Patients Vaccinated at Various British Institutes

London Vaccine Institution[27]	Vaccinated by Inoculations in Metropolis	
	In 1815	9,893
	From Beginning of Institute	28,887
	Vaccinated by Inoculators in County	
	In 1815	16,457
	From Beginning of Institute	324,007
Hospital for the Small-pox, for Inoculation and for Vaccination, at Pancras[5]	Vaccinated Jan. 19, 1799– Jan. 1, 1819 at	43,394
Vaccine Society[28] City of Northern Liberties District of Southwark	Vaccinated by Physicians of Society 1809–1817	10,633
Small-pox Hospital, London[29]	Vaccinated Jan., 1799–1805	13,715

ties, it was incapable of producing this change upon the human frame which is requisite to render it unsusceptible of the variolous contagion: so that it became evident a person might milk a cow one day, and having caught the disease, be forever secure; while another person, milking the same cow the next day, might feel the influence of the virus in such a way, as to produce a sore or sores, and in consequence of this might experience an indisposition to a considerable extent; yet, as has been observed, the specific quality being lost, the constitution would receive no peculiar impression.[4]

As a result of Dr. Jenner's encouraging report and pursuit of this valuable experiment of nature, many physicians (Table 6) began to practice vaccination in the early nineteenth century. Table 7[5] shows the favorable response of vaccination in terms of smallpox patients registered at one London Hospital in periods before (1779–1790) and after (1799–1818) the advent of vaccination. The practice spread quickly from England to France and other European countries, and to the new United States of America. Societies, and vaccination institutions devoted to this remarkable procedure, as well as special hospitals flourished early in the nineteenth century, and included such agencies as:

National Vaccine Establishment of London
Medical Committee for the Vaccine Inoculation at Paris
Vaccine Society of London
Cow-pox Institution (Dublin)
Kine-pox Institution (Boston)

Dispensary for Infant Poor and Cow-pox Inoculation
Vaccine Institution (Edinburgh)
Central Vaccine Society of Paris
Vaccine Pock Institution
Vaccine Establishment (Bengal)
Philadelphia Vaccine Institution

Table 7
Deaths Attributable to Smallpox*

	Registered at Pancras Hospital for the Small-pox, for Inoculation and for Vaccination†	*Registered by Parish Clerks of London (General bills of Christenings and Burials)*
1779–1798 Before Vaccination	1867	36,189
1799–1818 Since Vaccination	814	22,480

*From J. C. Wachsel, London Med. Repository, "Monthly Journal and Review" 11 (1819) 257.[5]
†A total of 43,394 persons vaccinated from January 19, 1799 to January 1, 1819.*

Gloucester Vaccine Association

Broad Street Vaccine Institution

Institution for the Gratuitous Inoculation of Cow-Pox (Edinburgh)

Vaccination Establishment, Berlin (Impfinstitut)

Special hospitals for vaccination and treatment of this disease included the Small-pox Hospital in London, and the Hospital for the Small-pox, for Inoculation and for Vaccinations at St. Pancras. The large numbers of inhabitants in selected British communities vaccinated for smallpox during the early nineteenth century are shown in Table 7. It required about five to six years, after Jenner's original promulgation of the vaccination procedure, for a noticeable reduction in smallpox mortality to be noted in Britain. This was a much happier response than that observed almost a century before after the introduction of inoculation (as opposed to vaccination with cowpox), because the former procedure actually enhanced mortality attributable to smallpox. An example of the former, adverse effect was provided by Blane in 1820 who reported[45]:

The Ratio of Mortality Due to Smallpox Compared to Total Mortality

> From 1706–1720; 78 smallpox deaths in 1000 deaths
> Inoculation Introduced:
> From 1745–1759; 89 smallpox deaths in 1000 deaths
> From 1785–1798; 94 smallpox deaths in 1000 deaths
> Vaccination Introduced:
> From 1805–1818; 53 smallpox deaths in 1000 deaths

The optimistic prophesy of Blane[6] in July 1820 that "it is now matter of irrefragable historical evidence, that vaccination possesses powers adequate to the great end proposed by its meritorious discoverer, in his first promulgation of it in 1798, namely the total extirpation of smallpox," would require almost 158 years to be realized, worldwide. His prophesy was correct, but his basis for it—the "irrefragable historical evidence"—accumulated over a period of 20 years of vaccination was inadequate. The eradication of smallpox would eventually require not only improved vaccines prepared in modern twentieth century laboratories and the organizational cooperation of member states of the World Health Organization, but unique, constant, fast-reacting surveillance methods coordinated on an international scale. The early history of smallpox vaccination followed a course quite analogous to that followed in modern times for medical discoveries, the principal difference being only the rate of progression. Steps in this development of Jenner's discovery included

1. An observation by a trained and curious medical expert;
2. Experimental testing of the hypothesis;
    a. In Jenner's case, human testing,
    b. In modern times, animal testing precedes human testing.
3. Reporting of the discovery in widespread medical journals;
4. Confirmation by other medical experts;
5. Accumulation and analysis of statistics providing evidence of the treatment effectiveness;
6. Open publication and debate of the effectiveness of the discovery;
7. Reporting of toxic or adverse effects of the treatment;
8. Later commercial, mass production, or public health utilization of the technique.

It is noteworthy that the above stages not only reflect the patterns that are still followed in modern scientific medical developments, but they elucidate a modus operandi usually not seen prior to early nineteenth century medicine.

In earlier times, qualified investigators did indeed report experimental findings. However, accounts pertaining to Jenner's vaccination procedure illustrated certain early nineteenth century advances including 1) increased public debate in the journals, made possible only by the proliferation of medical journals in this period, 2) significantly increased reliance of statistical or quantitative evaluation of mortality and morbidity data and registries, and 3) an efficient and popular venture in preventative medicine approached by both medical and governmental bodies as a practice in public health.

Royal Command for Evaluation of Vaccination

The King of England commanded in 1807 that the Royal College of Physicians of London, and that the Royal Colleges of Surgeons of London, Dublin and Edinburgh inquire into the state of vaccine inoculation in the United Kingdom, to report their opinion(s) and observations upon the practice, upon the evidence which has been adduced in its support, and upon the causes which have hitherto retarded its general adoption.[7]

This they did, and Dr. Lucas Pepys, president of the Royal College of Physicians replied in a letter published in the *Medical and Physical Journal* in August, 1807. He concluded that

the College of Physicians feel that it their duty strongly to recommend the practice of vaccination. They have been led to this conclusion by no preconceived opinion, but by the most unbiassed judgment, formed from an irrestible weight of evidence which has been laid before them. For when the number, the respectability, the disinterestedness, and the extensive experience of its advocates, is compared with the feeble and imperfect testimonies of its few opposers; and when it is considered that many, who were once adverse to vaccination, have been convinced by further trials, are now to be ranked among its warmest supporters, the truth seems to be established as firmly as the nature of such a question admits; so that the College of Physicians conceive that the public may reasonably look forward with some degree of hope to the time when all opposition shall cease, and the general concurrence of mankind shall at length be able to put an end to the ravages at least, if not to the existence, of the small-pox.[6]

The verbosity of this positive assertion was typical of the times. Nonetheless, it officially sealed the fate of continued vaccination. The Royal College of Physicians of Edinburgh at the same year was also so markedly swayed by the benefit of vaccination that they spontaneously and unanimously elected Dr. Jenner an Honorary Fellow of their College — a mark of distinction which they very rarely conferred, and which they confined almost exclusively to foreign physicians of the first eminence.[6]

Opposition to Vaccination

As illustrated above the public acceptance and beneficial effects of vaccination were becoming widespread. Dr. James Moore, who was director of the National Vaccine Establishment, Surgeon of the Second Regiment of Life Guards, amongst other notable distinctions, published in 1817 *The History and Practice of Vaccination*. Reference was made in this book to the opposition group to vaccination, which was as well evident (Fig. 30) in many published articles in the first two decades of the nineteenth century. Moore referred to this opposition as

the reptile tribe of practice hunters, whether fluttering or creeping; the needy pamphleteers; wonder-mongers; and speech makers, each after his kind; who set themselves in opposition to vaccination either from lack of wit or from lack of money, and who, Heaven knows! are too gone for argu-

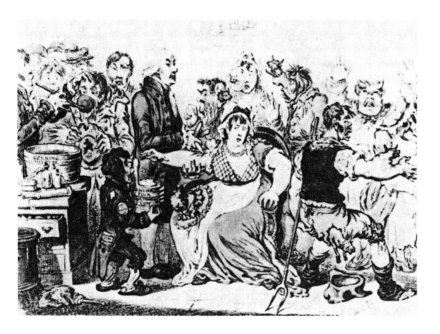

Fig. 30. "Cow Pock," an etching by the well-known early nineteenth century caricature artist, James Gillray, and printed in London in 1802. As illustrated in this caricature, vaccination with material from cows was a highly controversial procedure after its discovery and early exploitation. This scene is thought to represent the Small-pox and Inoculation Hospital at St. Pancras.

ment; yet on all that is venerable and respectable in our community for rank, intellect, or influence, we anticipate that they will produce a most solid and indelible impression in favour of the efficacy of this most brilliant discovery; a discovery, which, in the eyes of posterity will give greater eclat to this, our age, than the late tremendous conflicts of contending armies; the wondrous rise or fall of dynasties; or the upraising or upsetting of thrones.[8]

If such an emotional appeal can be considered a verbal effusion, then it was countered by Sir Gilbert Blane of London who asked in 1820 that physicians favor vaccination and he suggested "that the clamorous effusions of party are changing into the cool discussions of men of science."[9]

Nonetheless, failures of vaccination (and inoculation) in protection against smallpox, and aversion to this procedure were widely publicized. Although not antagonistic to this procedure, the well-known American physician, Dr. Benjamin Rush published an account in 1808 of the failure of this procedure, facts which he submitted for the "consideration of the enemies of vaccination, and the queries which follow them to the friends of free inquiry into medicine."[10] His case consisted of a sea captain who had been ill two days with an acute fever, attended with bleeding from his nose. The doctor had bled him twice, and had purged him freely. We concurred in directing a third bleeding. The next day an eruption appeared all over his body, which I suspected to be the small-pox. He said that was impossible, for that I had inoculated him, twenty-six years before, for that disease, and, as a proof of it, showed me the mark usually left by the pustule on the arm; also two distinct pock-marks upon his leg. To prevent a mistake in this business I called upon his mother, who assured me, that he had the usual fever and number of eruptions from inoculation....[10]

It was recognized, as reported by a New York physician, Dr. John D. Gillepsie, that

even in the most healthy children, it is sometimes necessary to vaccinate two or more times, owing either to the virus of the infection being impaired, or more probably to some other action going on at the time in the system of the child. It may also happen from an improper mode of performing the operation.[11]

The *Philosophical Magazine* in 1811 also reported (National Vaccine Establishment Report) a series of cases of failure of vaccination to prevent smallpox, including as one victim the Honourable Robert Grosvenor, third son of the Earl of Grosvenor. This case and the others proved to be mild cases, and it was suggested that

the general advantages of vaccination are not discredited by the instances of failure which have recently occurred, the proportion of failures still remaining less in number than the deaths which take place from the inoculated small-pox.[12]

Dr. John Ring, member of the Royal College of Surgeons in London, reported[13] in 1815 of an interesting case in which smallpox twice struck a young girl who had previously been vaccinated, and the editors of the journal containing his report conceded that such an incident proved "the impossibility of reducing the laws of contagion to a system." Other brief case reports on the occurrence of smallpox after vaccination were also published.[9,14,15]

The aversion to vaccine inoculation existed not only in Britain, but in continental Europe as well. One antagonist was Dr. Marcus Herz of Berlin, who was "one of the most respectable physicians of Germany, and justly celebrated by several of his publications."[16] Herz's memoir, published in *Hufeland's Medical Journal* at the turn of the century, was entitled "On the Brutal Inoculation, and its Comparison with the Human Inoculation." He protested the introduction of "a brutal (animal) poison into the human constitution." A complainant in London published his antagonistic 76 page memoir, "A Conscious View of Circumstances and Proceedings Respecting Vaccine Inoculation" in 1800. This author, criticized for his anonymity in the *London Medical Review*,[17] claimed that the cowpox with its alleged contagion, had never affected the stately ox, the maiden heifer, or even the sucking calf. Neither, as far as my inquiries have gone has any suit ever yet been instituted by the lordly bull against his lady cow for her impurities: nor have the swine, so prone to disease eruption, been heard to grunt out one single complaint on the alarming occasion; but found contentedly to swill their wonted portions of whey and butter-milk in snorting gratulations.

This anonymous author questioned when he saw

an establishment (vaccination with cowpox vaccine) start up like a mushroom, and hears that a whole regiment has been punctured, and probed, and threaded with cow matter, he looks about him with astonishment, and his only conjective is, what may come next?

Dr. John Ring of London published a lengthy rebuttal to the earlier account of Dr. Rowley, who itemized many failures of the vaccination procedure. An exaggerated testament by Dr. Rowley of the vaccination controversy was presented in an 1807 issue of the *Medical and Physical Journal*:

I have been in some vaccine storms; and have had the buttons torn off my coat, cloth and all, to convince me of the great and infallible excellence of cow-pox. I have seen some few of the vehement vaccinators redden like a flame with fury; the lips quivering, the eyes starting out of the head, with flashing streams of fire; the mouth foaming, and tongue pouring forth a torrent of hard words, like a thunder storm, — the fist clenched like a pugilist, ready to accompany the violent wrath with other knock-down arguments.[18]

There is no doubt that there were many reasons for the cowpox vaccine to fail on occasion. Imperfect vaccine, and vaccination of subjects who were already in an early, nonsymptomatic stage of smallpox, were probably responsible for many reported cases of failure of vaccination. Some authors, such as Dr. Samuel Akerly of New York, assumed a moderate view in 1809, in testifying

though, in general, I am an advocate for vaccination, I would not smother the accounts which militate against it, and which are probably more numerous than the public are aware of, lest, by so doing, we rest our hopes in a false security. The object of such a proceeding would be to weigh the evidence of opposing facts, and strike a balance, to prevent running into extremes; neither to attempt to make this temporary residence of mankind a paradise, by annihilating disease, nor with Moselay and his chosen few, sword in hand, to attack the temple of Vaccina, and, like Mohomet and his followers to rush to battle with enthusiasm and madness.[19]

Reports in *The Eclectic Repertory and Analytical Review of Medicine and Philosophy* of 1811 attest to some of the factors affecting the vaccination controversy.

In truth, vaccination has had to struggle, not only against the indefatigable activity of avowed opponents, but also against the treacherous manoeuvres of pretended friends, and the misguided zeal of injudicious partisans ...

> It must also be remembered, that the general practice of vaccination is injurious to the pecuniary interests of the profession; and therefore, the patronage bestowed upon it by them is a most honourable proof of the candour and disinterestedness of the profession at large.[20]

Controversies to vaccination were waged in many countries soon after Jenner's technique was exported from Britain. In France, Dr. C. Laurent described the ongoing controversy in Germany, originally attested by George-Frederic Krauss in his 552 page volume, *Die Shutzpockenimpfung* in 1820.

> En vain les détracteurs de la vaccine voudraient profiter des moindres circonstances pour recommencer leurs attaques, et faire prendre pour des vices réels quelques légères imperfections qui tiernent au défaut de soin ou de méthode dans l'application de ce préservatif; en vain ils voudraient ouvrir des asyles pour priver de ses bienfaits la génération présente et celle à venir; la raison l'emportera sur les préjugés, et le moment n'est pas éloigné où cette précieuse decouverte pourra jouir du triomphe le plus complet.[21]

Vaccination was introduced into India in 1802 and was warmly encouraged there by the British government. Much aversion was seen to the introduction of Jenner's method there, because of

> a hatred to all innovations, ... a rumour (that) this was a design of the English to affix an indelible mark on certain persons: and that all males so impressed were, when they grew up, to be forced into the military service, and the females to be concubines.[22]

Further, resistance existed because the Hindus "had always considered the small-pox as a dispensation from a goddess named Mahry Umma; or rather that the disease was an incarnation of this deity into the person infected."[22] Thus, vaccination was first submitted to only by the Christians in India.

Aversion to vaccination with the cowpox vaccine was also notable in the new United States of America, shortly after Jenner's technique was introduced there by the respected Benjamin Waterhouse. Waterhouse was an intellectual, British-trained physician practicing in Boston. He had been appointed, at the age of 28, as Harvard's professor of the theory and practice of physic, in 1783. Waterhouse first described vaccination in 1799 in the *Boston Colonial Sentinel*, and strongly indorsed Jenner's method although he had not tried it himself. This was an ironic proposal from a man who had earlier advised "Let us leave the flowering path of speculation for the more arduous one of experiment," in his historical, 1792 book, *The Rise, Progress, and Present State of Medicine*, published in Boston.[23] However, Waterhouse soon industriously experimented with Jenner's method of vaccination after he received in July 1800 some threads of cowpox virus matter in a glass-stoppered bottle from Dr. Haygarth of Bath, England. The vitality of this virus sample, shipped from England, must be questioned. Nonetheless, Waterhouse quickly proceeded to vaccinate his own four children and various domestic helpers in his home. He became a fanatical propagandist and crusader of the vaccination procedure[24,25] as well as a controller of early distribution in America of vaccine arriving in glass vials from England.[26] The opposition to vaccination rapidly arose from several sources in the United States, for mostly the same reasons as it appeared in Britain. Bitter opposition came from the church which condemned, in principle, the introduction of noxious matter from diseased animals into humans as against God's will. Further opposition arose from physicians who were ignorant, nonbelieving, or jealous, and from variolation specialists (of the older inoculation procedure) whose livelihood was threatened. Owners of profitable smallpox hospitals were adverse to Jenner's discovery because their income was threatened, and the public resented accidents in the use of vaccination.

Methodology of Vaccination

In the early nineteenth century the methodology of vaccination was subject to considerable experimentation and debate. Indeed, even in modern times prior to the 1970's when smallpox vaccination was discontinued as a public health procedure, the method and type of vaccine (fresh calf lymph virus, purified and dried calf lymph virus, virus grown in chick embryo membrane, etc.) had varied and been subject to variable interpretation. We now know that initial vaccination against smallpox (i.e., prior to the very recent eradication of this disease) should be given between 12 and 24 months of age, unless the child were in an endemic area, because earlier vaccination reactions may be inhibited by placentally transmitted maternal antibodies. There are different types of normal reactions to the vaccina virus, which relate to the degree of immunity previously present in the patient vaccinated. These include 1) the most typical or "primary vaccinia" reaction (8-4 day maximal response; 10-12 cm areola; vesiculation and scar production), showing no previous immunity, 2) the accelerated or "vaccinoid" response (4-7 day maximal response; 4-6 cm erythema; vesiculation and smaller scar formation), showing partial immunity, and 3) the "immediate" reaction (8-72 hour maximal response; 1-2 cm erythema; no scar produced), showing high degree of immunity.

These variable responses which may occur normally, the variable and unreliable techniques and vaccine used by the early workers, and the lack of understanding of immunologic principles by physicians practicing in Jenner's time accounted for the early debate on methods.

Dr. George Gregory, physician to the Hospital for Small-pox and Vaccination at St. Pancras, published his "Cursory Remarks on Small-pox as it Occurs Subsequent to Vaccination," in 1823.[30] He felt that

> as a pathological principle, that the occurrence of small-pox, subsequent to vaccination, is dependent upon the intensity of the vaccine influence, as primarily exerted; and they lead to the belief, that the appearance of the cicatrix (scar) may be taken as a measure of that intensity.

Most other early workers also placed great importance on the scar, and Gregory was at least partially correct; there is a parallelism between 1) an observed smallpox reaction in the nineteenth century and the previous vaccine response and 2) the analogous reaction between previous immunity and the vaccine response as observed on patients in modern times, as described above. Gregory concluded in 1823 that vaccination did "not appear to lessen the violence, or shorten the duration, of the first or eruptive stage of fever, which is generally as severe, and even sometimes severer and longer in its duration than that of the casual confluent small-pox," but that it modified, by reduction, the progress of inflammation in the various eruption.[30]

Jenner outlined his recommended procedure of vaccination carefully:

> the vaccine fluid be taken, for the purpose of inoculation, from a perfect pustule on some early day of its formulation; I prefer the 5th, 6th, 7th, 8th and (if the efflorescence is not far advanced beyond the margin of the pustule) the 9th.[31]

Dr. Henry Dewar of Edinburgh, offering "practical inferences and observations" on vaccination, suggested

> In vaccination, the governing principle, which ought always to influence the surgeon, is to infect his patient most thoroughly with the virus. Little is to be feared from any excess of the vaccine fever; but an imperfect constitutional infection may produce a false security, and may diminish or frustrate the benefit expected from the operation. When three or more vesicles have been excited, lymph may be taken from this subject. But it is prudent always to leave two complete vesicles to pass through their course untouched....
>
> The prudent will not only avoid the perils proceeding from negligence and cold indifference, but will also eschew the practice of a most zealous clergyman of the Methodist presuasion, whom I once saw operate.
>
> This worthy man grasped his lancet firmly, but not after the fashion of surgeons. He continued alternately taking lymph from one infant, inserting it into another, and expounding his doctrine. A moment's pause occurring in his discourse, I seized the opportunity, and, to stop a work of super-vaccination, asked, "How many punctures he deemed necessary?" He proceeded with fluency, "So innocent is the lymph, so transitory its workings, and so lasting its effects, that, be assured, you cannot pour too much into the flesh."—In pronouncing these words, he impressed the epithets on his hearers with an elevation of the voice, and on the child with a depression of the lancet, who shrieked at each gesticulation. Yet the mother, who would have been infuriated had a surgeon extorted such screams, looked quite placidly at her revered pastor; being inwardly convinced, that all the pains taken and given by him, would, in some mysterious way, do good to her suckling.—As surgeons cannot expect to meet with the same indulgence, they are recommended to be more merciful in their mode of operating.[8]

Other refinements of vaccination were described,[32] as well as the character of the induced areolae, which sometimes were quite large.[33] An account of women themselves propagating smallpox during an outbreak in 1816 in Warminster, England, was unhappily described by one Dr. John Hoare.[34] He reiterated how "the women themselves propagated the disease with stocking needles, and soon spread it over the place." The women, panicked by the current smallpox epidemic, used the dangerous inoculation technique (of smallpox matter), which had been abandoned by most of the physicians for the vaccination procedure, known to be less dangerous.[34]

Physicians in Milan, Italy, such as Dr. Sacco, submitted "cow-pock matter" from Milanese cows for testing in England, whereupon it was observed that English patients at the Vaccine Institution responded similarly as they would have to vaccine prepared from British cows.[35] Dr. Sacco, interested in repeating the experiments of Jenner, went to great trouble to gather material from infected cows in Italy. When he finally found a group of infected beasts, he wrote,

> Although the pustules were already large and prominent, they did not yet appear to me sufficiently mature to yield the matter I wanted. As the cows were that day to go forward on their way to Milan, I found myself under the necessity of following them to their first halting-place, in order to examine them again next day. I walked out at an early hour to the meadow where they were at pasture. I examined the pustules, which appeared to me to be now arrived at maturity. They were lucid, and of a pale red colour, with a brown spot in the middle more depressed; and I thought this a favourable moment to collect the matter, which, through the assistance of the herdsmen, I was easily enabled to do by repeatedly soaking a thread in it.[35]

To improve the methodology associated with vaccination, Dr. James Bryce of Edinburgh suggested in 1802 a novel method of preserving vaccine matter. He proposed

> To have a small phial made for the purpose, having a long stopper which is ground at the upper part, so as to fit the mouth of the phial as exactly as possible, and that part of it which is within the phial is formed into square surfaces which are numbered. Upon these squares the virus is lodged, and when dry, is, with the stopper, put into the phial, where it is very completely secured from the action of the external air.[37]

Vaccination for Diseases Other Than Smallpox

Not surprisingly, success in preventing the dreaded smallpox by vaccination enticed early nineteenth century physicians to experiment with vaccination for other maladies. Dr. Valli of Constantinople inoculated himself with the plague in order to ascertain whether the vaccine prevented that disease. He used a mixture of variolus and pestilential (plague) virus, but unfortunately became infected with the plague.[37,38] It was claimed in *The*

Philadelphia Medical Museum of 1805 that a great number of persons in Constantinople had been vaccinated "to preserve themselves from the plague."[39]

Dr. John Archer of Maryland, after treating six or eight patients with the hooping-cough by vaccination, claimed that "of two formidable diseases, to which the human race are liable, the smallpox and hooping-cough, the first is prevented and the latter is cured by vaccination."[40] Others suggested, on the basis of case histories, that constipation was cured by vaccination,[41] but that vaccination afforded no protection against chickenpox.[42]

Further International Spread of Vaccination

As described above the exploitations and practical development of vaccination with cowpox matter was undertaken initially in Britain, mainly following the experimentation and early reports of Jenner. However, the earliest known published paper specifically referring to cowpox-induced protection against smallpox was a German report, published by an unnamed author, and appearing in 1769 in the weekly journal, *Allgemeine Unterhaltungen*. According to the editor of *The Philosophical Magazine* in 1803,[43]

> the above account affords another proof of the little dependence to be placed upon physicians in the application of facts to practice; and the more glaring they are, it seems, the more heedless, or even stupid, they have been in some instances, as in the present case. It now appears that the cow-pox prevails not only in the western countries of England, where the farmers discovered that their servants or themselves were exempted from the smallpox by having had cow-pox; but the same disease and the same fact of exemption were also known in other English countries; in Ireland, in Holstein, in Denmark, in many parts of Germany and even near Gottingen, in Switzerland, and in the Milanese. Nay, as long ago as 1769, the German journalists announced these facts, and the advantages over the small-pox.

This German author stated in 1769 that

> I must, however, remark, that in this country (Gottingen) those who have had the cow-pock are fully convinced that they are secured from the infection of the common small-pox, as I myself, on carefully inquiring into this circumstance, have often heard.[43]

After Jenner's reports and obvious success with vaccination, it did not take long for physicians outside of Britain to attempt this procedure. In many cases this was done by British physicians who traveled to the continent or abroad. In Valetta (Malta), Drs. Marshall and Walker introduced vaccination prior to January 21, 1801, indicating

> we have had the happiness to arrest the destroying progress of the smallpox, which has raged very much, and has been very mortal at Minorca and

Malta, and on board the fleet. The Minorgueens, who at first received the vaccine inoculation cautiously, are now very happy, and it is generally adopted among them. At Malta, the most complete success has attended us.[44]

In another letter, also dated in early 1801,[45] Dr. De Carro wrote to Dr. Jenner, indicating successful use of vaccination in Bohemia, Moravia, and the Venetian States, and stating:

> The German physicians are so perfectly convinced of the advantages of this inoculation, that they have printed a short and popular exhortation to the people, which has been put into the hands of all clergymen, who are ordered to deliver a copy of it to the father and godfather of every child who is brought to church to be christened.[45]

In Moravia the young nobleman, Count Francon Hugues de Salm, encouraged vaccination by offering two prizes, for the two Moravian physicians who were tTo inoculate the greatest number of children in one year.

In 1802 vaccination had gained ground in Spain; and Dr. Piguillem reported that over 7,000 persons were inoculated with cowpox in 1801–1802.[46] It was reported[20] in 1811 that manuals of vaccination in Chinese and Polish languages had been prepared, and it was said (incorrectly) that success with vaccination had been astonishing in the East Indies, and that "the numbers who have been vaccinated are such, that, in the settlements of Bombay, smallpox was said to be altogether exterminated." In Ceylon, vaccination was introduced in August, 1802, and Dr. Christie claimed that

> the number of vaccinated patients ... (vaccinated between August 1802 and June 30, 1806 amounted) to 47,523; and if, agreeably to a moderate calculation which I formerly made, not more than one-half of the inhabitants of this island escaped natural small-pox, and of the half that had it, one-third died, we may, without over-rating the benefits of vaccination, fairly estimate, that of the 47,523 patients who have been inoculated in the island (Ceylon), one-sixth of the whole, or 7,920, would have otherwise died of the small-pox, which, previous to the introduction of vaccination, was almost every year epidemic at Columbo, and many other parts of the island.[47]

It was claimed[48] in the 1814 Report of the National Vaccine Establishment that vaccination had "totally extinguished small-pox" in Ceylon and at the Cape of Good Hope, and that British Ambassador, Sir Gore Ouseley, had persuaded the Royal Family of Persia to adopt vaccination in Persia. Sweden,[48] India[22] and Denmark[9] practiced vaccination, and Waterhouse introduced the procedure to the United States, as described elsewhere in the present book. An astounding 2,671,662 persons had been vaccinated in France by 1817, and 200,000 people in Amsterdam by the same year.[49] In South America vaccination was also introduced during the first decade of the nineteenth century. Don Francisco de Salazar, who was a deputy to the Spanish Cortes, claimed that during his stopover in Peru on his way to London, that vaccination had been practised with so much energy and success in Lima, that, for the last twelve months, there had occurred, not only no death from, but no case of, small-pox; that the new-born children of all ranks are carried as regularly to the vaccinating house, as to the font of baptism; that the smallpox is entirely extinguished all over Peru; nearly so in Chili; and that there has been no compulsory interference on the part of the government to promote vaccination.[45]

The pattern of decreasing incidence of smallpox, followed by later outbreaks of the disease was to be observed worldwide until its total eradication in the 1970's.

Chapter VI

Medicine in the New United States of America

"The patient ... sometimes gets well in spite of the medicine."
Thomas Jefferson, 1807.

Although novel contributions to the development of Western medicine originating from the new United States in the early nineteenth century were slight by European standards, the new continent provided a milieu which would ultimately overshadow the latter in medical progress.

The invigorating environment in 1800–1825 was characterized by massive westward expansion of the new nation, a generally expanding economy interrupted only by short periods of financial depression, and a great population increase. The country was governed successively by Presidents Adams, Jefferson, Madison, and Monroe, and passed through the birth and demise of the Federalist Party control. In spite of growing pains associated with the earlier separation from Great Britain and a period of searching and seizure of U.S. ships by French and British warships, impressment of U.S. seamen by Britain, disruption of internal U.S. politics stemming from Napoleon's adventures in Europe, all finally resulting in the adoption of an 1807 Embargo Act of Jefferson and a declaration of war against Great Britain in 1812, the United States grew and solidified its nationalistic spirit. By 1815 it had again renewed close relations with Great Britain following the Treaty of Ghent.

Geographically, the United States of America moved its capital city to the undeveloped marshland of Washington, D.C. The Appalachian Mountains, which previously had limited the colonies to the narrow eastern continental seaboard, ceased to be a barrier for westward mobility (Figure 31), and by 1816 the population literally spilled westward beyond the mountain range, creating many new states and territories. The Lewis and Clark expedition, initiated by Thomas Jefferson, explored the territory obtained by the Louisiana Purchase, as well as regions along the Missouri River and finally the Rocky Mountains and Pacific seacoast. A complete doubling of area of the United

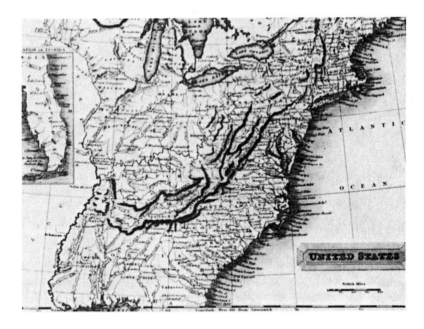

Fig. 31. The new United States of America. By 1823 the Appalachian Mountain Range had ceased to be a barrier to westward mobility.

States occurred during the initial 25 years of this century. Use of the Erie Canal, the development of turnpikes by enterprising businessmen, and the proving in 1807 of the economic success and reliability of the steamboat by Robert Fulton, all helped facilitate transportation and communication.

The early Americans increased in numbers dramatically, as attested by a census revelation of 5,300,000 inhabitants in 1800 (of whom 1,000,000 were Negroes, nine-tenths of which were enslaved), to 7,239,881 in 1810, and 9,638,453 in the total of 22 states in 1820.[2] Most of these Americans lived in the country; in 1830 the rural population was calculated at 91.3 percent. This was a nation of farmers and the large increase in manufacturers and industrial workers did not occur until later in the nineteenth century. Depending upon their location, the farmers depended on cotton, tobacco or rice crops (south and southwest), and wheat, corn, cattle, hogs, lumber, or other farm commodities (middle states). The farms of the New England states in the north were not prosperous, and commerce, cod and whale fisheries were of importance in the north in the early 1800's.[2, 3]

Thus, it was within the context of the above factors that practitioners of medicine, whether they were graduates of the elite medical schools of Western Europe, trained entirely by apprenticeship in the new United States of America, trained in newly established American medical schools, or quacks, found their work. Within the cities of Philadelphia, Boston, New York and a few other urban centers, medicine was practiced by the most sophisticated doctors of the nation, but in the majority of rural communities and farms, a lack of academically trained physicians was commonplace.

General State of Health in U.S.A., 1800

At the conclusion of the eighteenth century general health conditions and hygienic standards were extraordinarily low by today's standards, and the risk of dying at a young age was quite high in early America. The diseases, treatments, and risks were quite similar to those present in Europe at that time, and the similar health statistics in America, a new nation with only a small number of formally trained physicians compared to Europe, were attributable to the lack of real benefit provided by trained physicians in either location. At the time of the American Revolution, the average life expectancy was but 34.5 years for men and 36.5 years for women. As shown in Table 8, which presents the distribution of death by age for Charleston, Baltimore, New York, Boston, and London, England for 1818, 1819, or 1820,[4] close to 50 percent of deaths occurred prior to age ten. Infectious diseases were rampant, and typhoid, diptheria, malaria, measles, tuberculosis, cholera, and dysentery were omnipresent. Smallpox and yellow fever were periodic scourges, the latter disease decimating ten percent of the population of Philadelphia in 1793.

Table 8
Distribution of Death Age for Various Cities, 1818, 1819, or 1820
(Twelve month period)*

Ages	London England	Charleston SC	Baltimore MD	New York NY	Boston Mass.
Under 1 year			621	847	180
From 1 to 2	(Under 2)4779	(Under 3) 305	252	306	91
2 to 5	1771		129	188	41
5 to 10	826	(3–10) 84	147	103	38
10 to 20	631	61	291	157	49
20 to 30	1577	188	357	390	125
30 to 40	1990	156	191	383	94
40 to 50	2025	101	117	316	72
50 to 60	1913	78	71	200	55
60 to 70	1600	59	39	135	45
70 to 80	1230	20	35	93	33
80 to 90	666	27	27	45	16
90 to 100	144	9	9	10	—
Over 100	1	4	1	3	—

*Compiled from "The Eclectic Repertory and Analytical Review, Medical and Philosophical," 10 (1820) 278–290.[2]

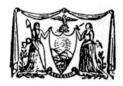

By GEORGE CLINTON, Governor of the State of New-York,
(L.S.) General and Commander in Chief of all the Militia, and
Admiral of the Navy of the Same :

A PROCLAMATION.

WHEREAS by the Statute entitled "An Act to prevent bringing
"in and spreading of INFECTIOUS DISTEMPERS in this
"State," it is enacted "That all Vessels of whatever kind
"they may be having on board any Person or Persons infect-
"ed with the YELLOW FEVER or any other contagious Distemper,
"or coming from any places infected with such contagious Distemper
"shall not come into any of the Ports or Harbours of this State, or
"nearer the city of New-York than the Island commonly called Bed-
"low's Island:" And whereas it is represented to me that the City of
Philadelphia is now infected with a contagious Distemper; where-
fore I DO by these presents strictly forbid and prohibit all Vessels
coming from Philadelphia aforesaid, and all other vessels coming
from any other place infected with any contagious Distemper, or
having on board any Person or Persons infected therewith from entering any of the Ports of this State, or to approach nearer to the City of
New-York than the said Island called Bedlows Island; And I do further hereby direct all Vessels coming from Philadelphia aforesaid or o-
ther place infected with such contagious distemper to perform Quaran
tine opposite the said Island and below the point of Governors Island
until such Vessel shall be duly discharged; And that no person
or Persons whomsoever, nor any Goods or Merchandize whatsoever
coming or imported in any such Vessel are to come or be brought on
shore or unloaded or put on board any vessel within this State, until the
Vessel so performing Quarantine shall be duly discharged as aforesaid, as every person offending in the premises will answer the same
at their peril. And I do also further enjoin and require the Branch
Pilots of this State and their deputies to be vigilant and attentive in
the performance of the duties required of them by the above recited
act conformably to the directions heretofore communicated to them.

GIVEN at the City of New-York under my Hand and the
Privy Seal this thirteenth day of September in the Seventeenth year of the Independence of the said State.

GEO : CLINTON.

Fig. 32. Quarantine, 1793, of vessels transporting persons afflicted with yellow
fever, arriving to New York from Philadelphia. (Original on file at the National
Library of Medicine, Bethesda, Maryland).

Pursuant to this tragedy in Philadelphia, George Clinton, the first
governor of the State of New York, issued a proclamation banning vessels
transporting any person afflicted with yellow fever and arriving from
Philadelphia, then capital city of the United States, from entering the ports of
New York. This early quarantine, depicted in Figure 32, dictated that such
vessels must be restricted to Bedlow's Island off New York. Typhus fever,
spread by body lice which were common on the early Americans who seldom
bathed, and scabies, scrofula, and scurvy were frequent maladies. As shown
in Table 9, consumption (tuberculosis) accounted for 11–20 percent of total
deaths in leading American cities in 1823.[5] Stillborn infant death rates were
high and poor obstetrical practices accounted for a high mortality of postpartum mothers. Cancers, which in present times account for the second highest
percentage of deaths in America, after cardiovascular-cerebrovascular-related
deaths, accounted for less than one percent of deaths in 1823. This was largely

Table 9

Proportion of Total Deaths due to Selected Causes as Listed in 1823 for Various American Cities*

Reported Cause of Death	Boston (City)	New York (City + County)	Philadelphia (City + Liberties)	Baltimore (City)	Charleston (City)
Cancer	0.3%	0.3%	0.4%	0%	0.5%
Consumption	16	20	12	11	17
Fever (all types)	8	6	13	15	16
Old Age	3	4	2	3	7
Still Born	8	7	5	5	–
Total Deaths (all causes)	1154 deaths	3444 deaths	4600 deaths	2108 deaths	814 deaths

*Compiled from annual reports from city Boards of Health, in "The Phil. J. Med. and Phys. Sci." 8 (1824) 238.[5]

Table 10
Bill of Mortality[1] for Portsmouth, New Hampshire, 1818[2]

Complaint	Total Deaths	Complaint	Total Death
Abscess	1	Gangrene	1
Apoplexy	3	Haemorrhage	1
Atrophy	7	Herpes	1
Cholera	3	Hysteritis	1
Cancer	1	Intemperance	1
Consumption	22	Inflammation of the Bowels	1
Croup	2	Inflammation of	1
Dropsy	3	the Liver	
Dropsy of the Brain	5	Pneumonia typhodes	4
Diarrhoea	1	Scrofula	3
Erythema	1	Scirrhous Liver	2
Fever, typhus	21	Sudden	3
Fever, pulmonic	4	Old Age (77–92 yrs.)	11
Fever, puerperal	1	Unknown Diseases	6
Fever, inflammatory	1	Accidental	6
		Total	118

[1] *Compiled by John Thurston, M.D., London Medical Repository Monthly Journal and Review 12 (1820) 261.*[6]

[2] *This capital city of New Hampshire was occupied by 6,934 inhabitants in 1810.*

due to the young age of most Americans at the time of their death, usually caused by infectious disease, but differences in diagnostic capabilities, and perhaps lesser exposure to carcinogenic environmental factors in the early 1800's also contributed to this difference. A typical bill of mortality for this period in early America is shown in Table 10, which summarizes the alleged causes of death for the City of Portsmouth, New Hampshire for 1816.[6] Consumption and typhus fever together accounted for 36 percent of all deaths that year, which is probably a reasonably accurate figure due to the ease of diagnosis of these diseases. However, many other disease entities ascribed as a cause of death on this bill of mortality, such as "atrophy," "inflammatory fever," are now known not to be specific disease; diseases of this era were both characterized and treated on the basis of gross symptomology, their true causal agents not being understood in this pre-microbiologic time.

General State of Medical Practice in U.S.A., 1800

The first practice of medicine in a sophisticated manner on the North American continent began in Mexico, the Spanish being the first to come and organize medical schools and hospitals. An account of this early and interesting history of medicine, which begins with the founding of the first hospital in Santo Domingo in 1503, has been provided by Major.[7] The University of Mexico had established the first chair of medicine in North America in 1580, and

Spain had created eight universities on this continent prior to the founding of Harvard University by early settlers in 1636 in New England. Also in the west early missionaries contributed to the development of medicine. During the Franciscan Mission Period of Alta California (1769–1833) medical care was provided for both whites and Indians at the missions. Fourteen cesarean operations were performed in Alta California between 1772 and 1833, mostly upon deceased mothers, and primarily for the purpose of baptising a live infant for the glory of God — such infants always died and the performance of the operation was noted in the Burial Registers.[8]

On the eastern seaboard of North America medicine was originally practiced in a much more primitive fashion than in the nonrelated, early Western Spanish settlements. A single physician, Dr. Samuel Fuller, had landed with the Mayflower in 1620, and he served the colony until 1633 when he died of smallpox. Subsequent to his arrival, and for perhaps 175 years, medicine in the colonies and newly formed United States of America tended to be dominated by quackery, mystical and superstitious beliefs, home remedies, and medical care provided by ministers, magistrates, schoolmasters, local political leaders, planters in the southern colonies and physicians who generally possessed little or no training and no medical degree. Charlatans prospered in this period; one early nineteenth century historian reported:

> Quacks abound like Locusts in Egypt, and too many have recommended themselves to a full Practice and profitable Subsistence. This is the less to be wondered at as the Profession is under no Kind of Regulation. Loud as the Call is, to our Shame be it remembered, we have no Law to protect the Lives of the King's Subjects, from the Malpractice of Pretenders. Any Man at his Pleasure sets up for Physician, Apothecary, and Chirurgeon. No Candidates are either examined or licensed, or even sworn to fair Practice."[9]

Although a few qualified physicians trained in Western Europe emigrated to the colonies, they were very rare in relation to the total number of early settlers. The Indians in eastern North America continued to consider disease as an evil, supernatural malady which was best treated by singing and dancing, body painting, herbal remedies, fetishes, fires, bleeding, and counter-irritation, etc.[10] Prayer, fasting, heat, blood-letting, Indian remedies, and the widespread use of purging and emetics constituted the principal medical treatments of the early colonists. At the beginning of the War of Independence it is estimated that there were about 2,500–3,500 practitioners of medicine of which about 200–400 were doctors of medicine and 50 were graduates of the two medical schools then established in the colonies.[10-15] Medical schools had been founded at the College of Philadelphia in 1765 and at King's Medical College in 1768. Harvard Medical College was later to be established in Boston in 1782. The first hospital in the colonies was founded on Long Island in 1663.

As suggested by the quotation above, written by a scholar in the colonies, the people of the general public who were considerably less educated viewed the medical profession with a mixture of fear and contempt. In 1775 the people of Northampton County in Pennsylvania submitted a petition to the Assembly in Philadelphia requesting a law forbidding any "except those of established and unquestionable Reputation" to practice medicine or surgery "until he or they have first undergone an Examination before two or more skilful and judicious Physicians of the City of Philadelphia."[9] Dissatisfaction with the state of the art of medicine and the integrity of its practitioners was also expressed by the practitioners who overtly argued amongst themselves in the community, at the patient's bedside, and in the medical journals. Dr. Akerly of Philadelphia published the statement in 1808 in the *Medical Repository*:

> From the general want of information among this class of practitioners (i.e., those who are quacks and who employ inert remedies), we are inclined to despise most of their remedies even when known, as they appear to be given without discretion or a proper discrimination, by their exhibition in the various stages of different and opposite diseases. This want of attention to quack remedies, has no doubt retarded the progress of medicine. Dr. Rush enumerates it as such in his lecture on this subject.[16]

Thomas Jefferson, a man of many talents who was third president of the United States (1801–1809), and notable contributor to the development of paleontology, to scientific agriculture, to mechanical invention, to international diplomacy, and to architectural design, also had his logical views of medical practice in the early 1800's. Although not directly involved in medicine, Jefferson nonetheless read widely in medicine, collected a large section of medical treatises in his extensive library of 6,000 volumes, and actively corresponded with physicians about the status of science in relation to medicine. As reviewed by Hall,[17] Jefferson approached medicine with the same logical view as he approached all matters, and was deeply concerned about the health and physical well-being of Americans. Jefferson was critical of medicine partly because of his firm scientific conviction that any scientific inquiry must be based on observation and experiment, and that too many adventurous physicians substituted presumption for knowledge. He felt that the greatly diversified nature of clinical symptoms precluded the accurate assessment of a definite disease, and that an unknown disease could hardly be treated by a known remedy. In his design and establishment of the University of Virginia, Jefferson encouraged the inclusion of a school of medicine in this new institution, which was opened in 1825. Thomas Jefferson was also a strong proponent of the use of the new preventive vaccination for smallpox, just developed by Jenner and first used in the United States by Benjamin Waterhouse in 1800. He ordered the vaccination of Indians visiting the White House as a gift of the Great Spirit to all men,[17] and requested that Lewis and Clark take a supply of smallpox vaccine along on their explorations in order to vaccinate persons they contacted.

Those physicians who adhered to the allegedly scientific principle of basing conclusions upon careful observations, rather than hearsay, personal bias, or some of the classical treatments used in Europe in the early 1800's which were directly derived from Hippocrates, Galen, or Elsus, also succumbed to illogical thought processes. These fallacies commonly related to the lack of adequate control of observations or experiments, the neglect of spontaneous cures occurring in the presence of a remedy, and the fallacious assumption that a cure follows the application of a remedy; the remedy therefore has produced the cure; *post hoc, ergo propter hoc.*

Thomsonian Movement

As a result of general dissatisfaction on the part of the public with medical treatments and charlatans in the early 1800's, alternative and self-administered modes of therapy began to become popularized. The public was not blind to the lack of success of the heroic medical practices of blood-letting, purging, and blistering.[18] One such alternative mode of treatment, referred to today as the Thomsonian Movement, consisted of a system of medicine dependent upon use of botanical drugs. The originator of this method was Samuel Thomson (1769–1843), a self-made man who through his own frustration with the uselessness of heroic medicine and his inspiration by an old herbal "doctor" lady in New Hampshire taught himself about the use of roots and herbs. Thomson gave up farming in 1805 to become a traveling herb doctor and met with great success in parts of Maine, Massachusetts, and New Hampshire.[19] In 1811 Thomson organized followers of his system of botanical medicine into a society in Eastport, Maine. He published a "medical circular" in 1812 and patented his system in 1813. His circular, after several expansions, was published as a book (*New Guide to Health*) in 1822, which ultimately went through thirteen editions. It will not be surprising to see a fourteenth edition of Thomsonian medicine in modern times, in view of increasing popularity of folk-medicines and natural health foods! Thomson's system of medical therapeutics, described by Rothstein,[19] progressed through a series of "courses," which were numbered, contained a variety of botanical emetics and tonics, and correlated body heat with degree of health and food intake. Much of his advice was sound, particularly his rejection of the traditional and heroic practices of blood-letting, the use of blisters, and the use of arsenic (ratsbane) and other toxic agents. Thomson's view on bleeding is shown in his statement[20]:

> The practice of bleeding for the purpose of curing disease, I consider most unnatural and injurious. Nature never furnished the body with more blood than is necessary for the maintenance of health.... If the system if diseased, the blood becomes as much diseased as any other part; remove the cause of the disorder, and the blood will recover and become healthy as soon as any other part; but how taking part of it away can help to cure what remains, can never be reconciled with common sense...

The wide variety of botanical agents prescribed in Thomson's book included herbs and roots that were relatively well-known to the more traditional physicians of his day, such as hemlock, raspberry tea leaf, white pond lily, myrtle bush-bark or root, peach kernels, ipecac, etc. Thomson claimed originality for lobelia (Indian tobacco), although originality was refuted.[19] His uniqueness was in organizing the botanical agents into a publicized system, and imparting to his patients the proscription of harmful remedies used by the more traditional physicians. Eventually the Thomsonian movement became institutionalized as a state medical society (New York, 1835), and ultimately various botanical medical schools and infirmaries were developed in several U.S. states which had philosophic linkage with the Thomsonian movement. Dr. Richard Carter of Kentucky also published a book in 1825 advocating botanical prescriptions.[21] The Thomsonian Movement has been described in detail by Berman,[22] who re-published the following poem describing the virtues of Thomsonian medicine. This poem was originally published in 1834 in the heyday of Thomsonian popularity.

> The Grace, though silent, can instruction give!
> Disease has thousands slain; ten thousands art,
> (Falsely so nam'd,) has hurried to the grave!
> Merc'ry, the bane of life, is crowded down
> The infant throat, as if't were healing balm!
> Custom has led the way, and book-worms crawl
> Along the beaten track, nor once suspect
> The show of wisdom folly has contrived.
> Blind! — Leaders of the blind! lift up your eyes
> And seek for light, that leads from ruins brink!
> Your Calomel, and all your deadly drugs, reject!
> The world is wakening round you! Botanic
> Doctors (sounding the majesty of truth)
> Gain ground: the mercurial craft declines!
> Thick darkness flies before Thomsonian light,
> Bursting in glory on a long benighted world!
>
> (From preface to *The Thomsonian Recorder*, vol. II, Columbus, Ohio, 1834).

Another special system of medicine described as *homeopathy* was developed by Samuel Christian Friedrich Hahnemann, in Germany. This system, which was originated by Hahnemann's experiments in 1790, and which, like Thomson's system, proscribed the use of blisters, blood-letting, etc., advocated the use of special, very small doses of drugs. Homeopathy was transported to the United States in 1825 by the German, Hans Gram, and was later promoted widely by Constantine Hering in the new country. Thus, this system had not achieved importance in American medicine in the first quarter of the nineteenth century, but later became popular as a result of growing hostility toward conventional medical practices in early America. The Thomsonian and homeopathic systems of medicine were not the only ventures to create novel doctrines of medical therapeutics and practice in the early 1800's.

So many different systems had been promoted by this time that Thomas Jefferson claimed of seeing the systems of Hoffman, Boerheave, Stahl, Cullen and Brown "succeed one another like the shifting of figures of a magic lantern."[17] Although some systems such as the Thomsonian system were reactionary to the failures of traditional medical practices, many physicians were themselves reactionary to the proliferation of "systems medicine." Such physicians saw a natural conflict between a *system* approach versus clinical *experience*, and favored experience. Thus, one proponent of the experience school, Dr. J. Augustine Smith, said "It is our business to observe well, to observe long, and to observe all."[23,24] This advocation for observation in American medicine, as in Western Europe, was manifest in many ways. In clinical papers, such as published by Dr. Akerly of Philadelphia on the use of ergot or spurred rye in cases of delayed parturition, the reliance on observation was expounded[16]:

> The prejudices which you observe exist in Europe against the use of the Ergot, as being actively injurious or contemptible for its inactive qualities, I know to be totally unfounded. I have administered it to more than one hundred parturient patients, and I have never given it except in cases that threatened a difficult or lingering labour. I do not recollect a single instance in which it did not ultimately succeed, and I have generally been able to predict from the commencement of its operation, with tolerable accuracy, the period of delivery. This satisfactorily proves to me its active qualities. That it is not injurious you will have some reason to believe, when I assure you that I never lost a patient that I attended during her parturition, neither immediately, nor in consequence of sickness thereby induced; and that I have never had any case where the disorder could be traced to this source. I find it is more active when prepared by decoction than in powder; I therefore always prefer the former. It is much to be regretted that scientific physicians have generally held in contempt every medicine that quacks have been in the habit of administering. When we reflect that accident has given origin to the use of our most active medicines, and that we are indebted to empiricism for a knowledge of their most useful qualities, we certainly should neglect no opportunity of deriving aid to science from this source.

Other more exacting methods of observation were indeed being used in the early American states of medicine. As shown in the previous tables and in Table 11, the epidemiologic character of disease incidence was being quantitatively observed and published. Notably, a seasonal variation in death rates attributable to dysentery and infantile flux was observed in several American cities during the late summer months (1819–1820). As described by William Osler in 1897,[25] one of the most rigorous, impartial observationists and scientific note-takers on human pathology was Dr. M. Louis. Louis, a Frenchman trained in Rheims, Russia, and Paris had a profound influence on American medicine through his numerous pupils who practiced in America from 1830. However, he developed and practiced his system of accurate description and recording during the second decade of the nineteenth century and published in 1823 a memoir on perforation of the small intestines in acute disease, and

Table 11
Total Deaths by Month for Various Cities, 1819-1820*

	Charleston S.C.	Baltimore Md.	Philadelphia Pa.	New York N.Y.	Boston Mass.
January	65	124	192	250	57
February	52	116	195	223	52
March	61	143	259	199	55
April	60	169	214	226	50
May	97	135	204	196	56
June	85	121	259	207	33
July**	84	238	338	261	52
August**	145	316	432	460	94
September*	173	474	288	309	113
October	90	243	242	309	83
November	68	104	254	266	78
December	46	104	247	220	66

*Compiled from The Eclectic Repertory and Analytical Review, Medical and Philosophical 10 (1820) 278-290.[4]

**Diseases peculiar to warm season especially increased mortality to children ("dysentery and infantile flux")

others on croup in the adult, and cardiac disease, and in 1824 two memoirs on pathological anatomy of the stomach lining and one on pericarditis. Louis' 1825 volume on phthisis was very popular, and his later numerical analyses on the lack of benefit of blood-letting were of great significance in the early development of medical statistics.

The Journals and Distinguished Physicians, 1800-1825

The first medical journal to be published in America was the *Medical Repository*, which first appeared in July 1797. By 1807, seven journals were appearing in the United States, including the *Philadelphia Medical Museum* (1804), and the *Philadelphia Medical and Physical Journal* (1804). The famous *New England Journal of Medicine*, which today is one of the most prominent medical journals in international circles, began in Boston in 1812 under the name, *New England Journal of Medicine and Surgery and the Collateral Branches of Science*. These journals provided a popular forum for physicians in America who now had a place to report their interesting case histories, theoretical views on therapy, and empirical findings. Also, the historiography of American medicine, while not originating as late as 1800, acquired an importance in the medical field during the first decade of the nineteenth century, and American medical experiences in the Revolutionary War and Campaigns of 1812[26,27] as well as civilian medical progress were recorded.[28-31]

Prominent medical names abound in early America during the first

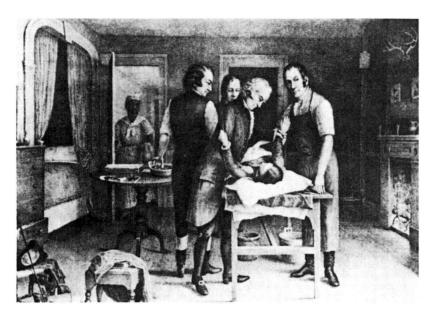

Fig. 33. Dr. Ephraim McDowell of the United States of America performed in a Kentucky cabin the first successful ovariotomy in 1809. Note the lack of anesthesia, lack of sterile procedures, and the slave in the background. (Original on file at the National Library of Medicine, Bethesda, Maryland.)

three decades of the 1800's, although their familiar ring is based perhaps as much upon their impact on the development of medicine in the pioneer environment of America as it is upon the originality of their contributions to medical science in the Western world. Such individuals included Dr. Daniel Drake, the prominent contributor to American medicine in the Western (i.e. Ohio) United States. Although many of his important works were published during 1841–1852, his earlier contribution on "The Climate and Diseases of Cincinnati" (1810), was notable, being the first medical writing of the West. William Beaumont (see chapter on digestive diseases), later to become a well-known investigator in American medicine with his 1833 and ultimately classic, *Experiments and Observations on the Gastric Juice and the Physiology of Digestion*, published his first brief account of his work in 1825 in the *Medical Recorder*. Dr. Ephriam McDowell (Figure 33) became the founder of U.S. abdominal surgery in 1809 when he performed the first successful oophorotomy in the small wilderness town of Danville, Kentucky. McDowell, who was trained by preceptorship in Virginia and later under various well-known doctors in Edinburgh, removed a 22½ pound ovarian tumor from a stricken lady during his initial classic ovariotomy, while concerned relatives and friends of the patient waited outside the cabin with rope in hand. He published an account of this procedure, along with several other similar cases he successfully carried out and these were widely acclaimed during the time of his practice.

Benjamin Winslow Dudley (1785–1870) was another prominent surgeon of this period, and was professor of anatomy and surgery at, and developer of Transylvania University at Lexington, Kentucky. Other prominent U.S. physicians and medical school professors in the early 1800's included William Shippen, Jr. (1736–1808), who was earlier associated with John Morgan (who held the first medical professorship in North America at The University of Pennsylvania), Dr. Adam Kuhn (1741–1817), Dr. Caspar Wistar (1760–1818), Dr. Philip Physick (1768–1837), and Drs. Samuel Bard, David Hosack, John Warren, James Jackson, and Valentine Mott. Dr. Benjamin Rush and Dr. Benjamin Waterhouse were particularly noteworthy. Rush was undoubtedly the most famous of U.S. physicians of Revolutionary times, and prior to his death in 1813 had as well been a signer of the Declaration of Independence, a crusader for hospitals for alcoholics, for free dispensaries for the poor, for public schools and higher educational facilities for women, and humane treatment for the insane. He is considered the first American psychiatrist. His last published book, *Medical Inquiries and Observations upon the Diseases of the Mind* was the first American psychiatry textbook, and was the only one in use for 70 years in the United States. Unfortunately, in spite of his great humanitarian ventures toward his society and immense reputation as a medical teacher, his overly-zealous use and indoctrination of students to use excessive bleeding and purging for most diseases without doubt contributed to the death of many patients. His theories of the organic-circulatory basis of many diseases, including mental disorder, have been described in many accounts,[7,32,33] and his policy of vigorous bleeding was in fact contested by some of his fellow practitioners. Thus, at the time of his death, he insisted on being bled, against the wishes of his attending physicians.

Of all the distinguished American physicians in the early 1800's Dr. Benjamin Waterhouse stands among the most elite. He was perhaps the best educated of such physicians, being trained in London, Edinburgh, and Leyden, and he helped establish Harvard Medical School. Waterhouse was appointed professor of the practice of physic at the University of Cambridge (which became the Harvard School of Medicine). His name is closely bound to the development of smallpox vaccination in the early United States, a medical advance of considerable importance. Smallpox was probably introduced into North America by the earliest settlers from Europe, since it was reported in various early accounts[34] that the Indians initially were of fine health in 1602, only later to become devastated periodically by epidemics of smallpox similar to those encountered on numerous occasions in the old world. The whites in America experienced the same problems with smallpox as they had in Europe, this disease constituting a major cause of their mortality. In 1721 approximately half of the population of Boston caught smallpox, and more than seven percent died.[12] At this time smallpox inoculation was introduced in America by Dr. Boylstone in Boston, through the interest of Cotton Mather, the preacher. This practice was highly controversial, and was forbidden at various times, but eventually statistics in 1753 seemed to indicate that smallpox contracted by inoculation was less apt to be fatal than if acquired in the natural way, as shown by the following result[35]:

Had smallpox the common way		Of these died	
Whites	Blacks	Whites	Blacks
5059	485	452(9%)	62(13%)

Received distemper by inoculation		Of these died	
Whites	Blacks	Whites	Blacks
1974	139	23(1%)	7(5%)

Inoculation continued to be practiced until 1798, when Jenner in England published his classic account on vaccination against smallpox, *An Inquiry into the Causes and Effects of the Variolae Vaccinae* (see chapter in the present book on smallpox). Jenner's method rapidly spread across England and across the Atlantic to the United States. Although there is some evidence that John Chichester, an Englishman in Charleston, South Carolina may have been the first to vaccinate a patient successfully in America in 1799,[36] credit is usually given to Benjamin Waterhouse, who successfully vaccinated four of his children on July 8, 1800. Thomas Jefferson officially sent a letter of congratulations to Waterhouse on Christmas day in 1800, on this successful vaccination, stating that "every friend of humanity must look with pleasure on this discovery, by which one evil more is withdrawn from the condition of man...."[37] Waterhouse's vaccine material had originated in England. The first genuine "kine-pock" which was developed from an American source was that obtained by Dr. Elisha North, who obtained his vaccine from a patient with cowpox in the spring of 1801. North, Waterhouse, and other early vaccinators against smallpox encountered opposition to their method of preventive treatment,[38] just as vaccinators in Europe had. The distinguished Dr. David Ramsay in America vigorously promoted smallpox vaccination after 1802, and in Charleston the establishment by Shecut of a vaccine institute and promotion of vaccination by a dispensary there helped popularize this procedure in the south.[39] Eventually Waterhouse became known as the "Jenner of America," and by 1810 at least one state, Massachusetts, had enacted legislation to require every community without a board of health to appoint individuals to organize and oversee vaccinations in their regions.[37]

Medical Education in the Early Nineteenth Century United States

Historical aspects of medical education in the United States during the 1800's have been well documented, including accounts presented in recent monographs on American medicine.[40,41] Accordingly, the purpose of the present account here is not to provide exhaustive details which can be found elsewhere, but rather to give an overview of early U.S. medical education.

Physicians were trained during the first quarter of this century predominately by an apprenticeship, which usually required three years at a cost of $100 per year, but occasionally required up to seven years, and triple that fee, depending upon the reputation of the teacher. The preceptor provided books and equipment, and issued a certificate to the apprentice upon successful completion of the course. The initial stage of training, termed "reading medicine with a doctor," included study of botany, physiology, materia medica (pharmacology), chemistry, pharmacy, clinical medicine, and anatomy which included dissection of animals and/or humans.[40] The second and final stage of training, termed "riding with the doctor," consisted of accompanying the doctor on house calls, in surgery, and in office clinical tasks such as blood-letting, wound dressing, etc. Because this system was not subject to any kind of quality controls or standardized examinations, or certification of preceptors, the quality of training was highly variable but usually poor. The medical students themselves were not competitively selected for medical training as they are today, and though some were undoubtedly talented and dedicated individuals, one former president of Yale University characterized them as the youth "that were too weak for the farm, too indolent for labor, too stupid for the law, and too immoral for the pulpit."[42] Rarely, trainees would travel to Europe for partial or complete medical education, and then return to practice in the United States. The apprentice system survived for a time not only because of a lack of licensing laws and formal medical schools in the United States, but also because preceptors found their trainees a source of added income and cheap labor. Further, the trainees would conveniently obtain a certificate to practice without strict examinations and without travel to distant centers of training. An example of a certificate to practice medicine, obtained by Dr. Daniel Drake from his preceptor in the early 1800's read as follows[43]:

> I do hereby certify, that Mr. Daniel Drake has pursued under my direction, for four years, the study of Physic, Surgery and Midwifery. From his good Abilities and marked Attention to the Prosecution of his studies, I am fully convinced that he is qualified to practice in the above branches of his Profession.
> Wm Goforth, Surgeon General,
> 1st Division Ohio Militia

The development of a medical licensing system in the early United States was a rather complicated phenomenon, interrelating with factors such as the clear inadequacy of the apprentice certificate, the increased number of newly-trained physicians, the rise in the number of new medical societies which promoted licensing, and the continual dissatisfaction by both patients and physicians in existing medical standards. While all of these variables contributed partly to regional legislation by licensing procedures and/or license requirements defined by medical societies, the development of licensing was sporadic. Statewide regulations, regulations for licensing within districts of states, and constant changes in regulations were encountered. It has been contended[40] that in the early 1800's the principal reason for development of medical licensing was an honorific one which provided selected physicians exclusive legal privileges that enhanced their community status, since the related variables mentioned above afforded little political clout to induce legislation. One of the legalistic outcomes of licensing legislation was the fact that only licensed physicians, in some regions, could sue for fees. It was only later in the nineteenth century that medical licensing became of significant importance in regulating medical practice.[40,44,45] In the first two decades of the nineteenth century professional regulation in medicine was inconsistent, and, according to Kett,[46] the determining factor was usually the level of social organization. In the older, larger cities on the eastern seaboard of the new United States, licensing regulation grew out of the medical societies or colleges which were patterned after the royal colleges in London. Further, stable organizations existed there which contributed to medical education, such as the first medical school at the University of Pennsylvania, and a circle of military surgeons possessing official medical designation and which were perpetuated after the American Revolution. One such surgeon was the U.S. Army Surgeon General, Joseph Lovell (1788–1836), who was the first Army physician to be appointed "Surgeon General" by Congress in 1818. (His collection of medical reference books later formed the basis of the Army Medical Library). In contrast, the licensing regulations in the newer and less populated regions of the United States were initiated from outside the medical professional circles, being instigated by legislatures in the newer states. Concurrently, with the increase in licensing regulations and general disfavor with the apprentice system, formal training of doctors increased. This initially took place mostly in private instruction classes, some of which formed the basis of later degree-granting medical schools. The steady increase in the number of regular medical schools in the first three decades of the nineteenth century is shown in Figure 34.[47] Many of these original schools later disappeared from existence. The number of U.S. graduates from formal schools, including private instruction classes also sharply increased by 1830 (Fig. 34). Although these schools occasionally had amongst their faculty distinguished physicians trained in Western Europe, they were mostly staffed by local practitioners who possessed very limited scientific credentials, and sought such professorships primarily for status-enriching and economic reasons.[46] There was an increasing trend to allow the diploma achieved from attendance at a medical school to serve as a license to practice. The medical societies played an integral role in both establishment of formal instructional programs, of medical schools as discrete institutions, as well as in the setting of specific criteria for licensure. Table 12 is a listing of medical societies which had been formed by 1825 in the United States of America. Many of these societies were short-lived.

Instruction in the newly formed medical schools consisted of didactic lectures covering basic medical sciences, the theory and diagnosis of diseases and surgical and medical therapeutics, and these lectures were supplemented by bedside training with a preceptor. Laboratory instruction was rare during

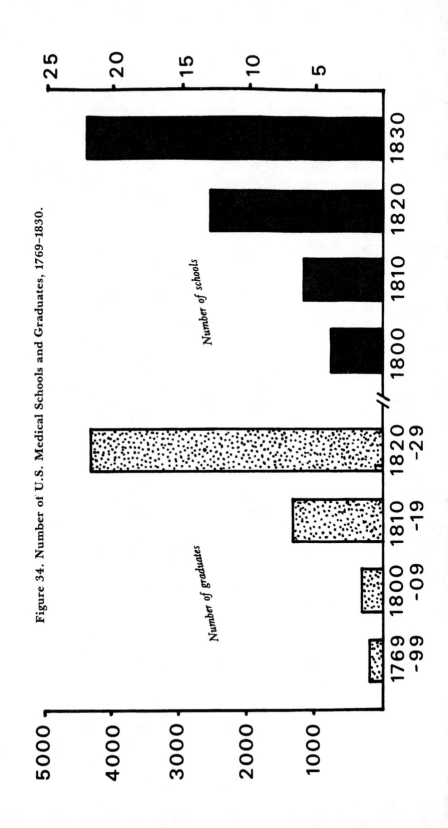

Figure 34. Number of U.S. Medical Schools and Graduates, 1769–1830.

Table 12

Founding Dates of Medical Societies
in Early America, through 1825[1]

Connecticut	1767–93	Various county societies founded
	1792	Connecticut State Medical Society founded
Delaware	1776	Medical Society of Delaware founded
District of Columbia	1817	Medical Society of the District of Columbia founded
Georgia	1804	Savannah City Society founded
	1822–28	Various local societies founded
Illinois	1817–25	Three medical societies incorporated by legislature
Indiana	1818, 1825	Incorporation of medical societies by legislature
	1817–35	One county and a state society founded
Kentucky	1802	Local society founded in Lexington; probably on this date, but before 1828.
	1819	Local medical society founded in Louisville
Louisiana	1817, 1820	In New Orleans medical societies founded for French and English speaking physicians
Maine	1810	Two local district societies of Massachusetts Medical Society founded (Maine at this time was part of state of Massachusetts)
	1820	Massachusetts State Medical Society founded
Maryland	1799	Medical and Chirurgical Faculty of Maryland founded as state society
	1815–25	Several local societies founded
Massachusetts	1781	Massachusetts Medical Society founded
	1804–25	Various local societies founded
Michigan	1819	Michigan State Medical Society founded
New Hampshire	1791	New Hampshire Medical Society founded
	1806–25	Various district societies founded
New Jersey	1807	Medical Society of New Jersey reorganized on a stable basis
	1790–1825	Numerous local societies founded
New York	1750–1825	Numerous New York and county societies founded
	1806	Medical Society of The State of New York founded

Table 12 (cont.)

North Carolina	1799	State society founded; suspended in 1804
Ohio	1812–24	Several state and district societies incorporated
Pennsylvania	1765	Philadelphia Medical Society founded; merged with American Philosophical Society in 1768
	1770	Local medical society founded in Philadelphia; discontinued in 1792
	1787	College of Physicians founded in Philadelphia
	1789	Philadelphia Medical Society founded
	1821–25	Local medical societies founded
Rhode Island	1812	Rhode Island Medical Society founded
South Carolina	1789–1808	Charleston and other local societies founded
Vermont	1804, 1813	Two county societies founded
	1814	Vermont State Medical Society founded
Virginia	1820	Richmond Medical Society founded
	1825	Local medical society founded

[1]*Data extracted from William G. Rothstein, "American Physicians in the 19th Century," The Johns Hopkins University Press, Baltimore, pp. 327–331, 1972. Numerous societies listed here were unstable and disbanded in subsequent years.*

the first two–three decades of the nineteenth century; Yale and Harvard medical schools were governed by conservative bodies which did not encourage scientific laboratories at this time, and actually resulted in formation of independent laboratories which were not even affiliated with the universities until later years.[48] Few American universities indeed had chairs in any of the basic sciences except mathematics and astronomy at the turn of the century although Benjamin Franklin (Fig. 35), David Rittenhouse, Joseph Priestley, John MacLean, and especially Benjamin Silliman favorably influenced the establishment of scientific faculties and basic science chairs in American universities in the early 1800's. It was generally considered that a complete medical faculty in 1815 would require seven persons, and that a minimum of four could constitute a faculty body sufficiently large to open a medical school. At Harvard University, for example, the early medical chairs and lectureships consisted of[49]:

> Hersey Professorship of Anatomy and Surgery (founded in 1783)
> > Held by John C. Warren, M.D. in 1816.
> Hersey Professorship of the Theory and Practice of Physic (1793)
> > Held by James Jackson, M.D. in 1816.
> Lectureship of Materia Medica and Botany (1815)
> > Held by Jacob Bigelow, M.D. in 1816.
> Lectureship of Midwifery (1815)
> > Held by Walter Channing, M.D. in 1815

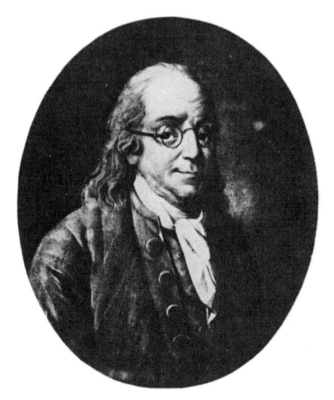

Fig. 35. Benjamin Franklin (1706–1790) founded the University of Pennsylvania, Philadelphia, which has the oldest medical school in the United States of America.

The inclusion of chemistry as a subject of medical study was open to some controversy, and was the cause of some debate at the University of Pennsylvania School of Medicine at the conclusion of the eighteenth century.[50] Nonetheless, Dr. John Morgan of Philadelphia was the first teacher of chemistry at America's oldest medical school at the University of Pennsylvania.

In an early history of Harvard Medical School described by Moore,[51] the procurement of adequate materials for anatomy instruction and dissection there as in other medical schools in the United States, was one of the problems which contributed to the colorful history of early medical training. Harvard was fortunate in 1816 in that it possessed an anatomical museum of numerous prized items of morbid anatomy, of wet preparations of healthy structure which were mostly injected, and of dry injected blood vessel preparations from different parts of the body.[49] It was claimed that the injected wet preparations of healthy structure were probably not exceeded in the United States in number or beauty! Wax representations of the ear, eye, and reproductive organs, specimens of urinary calculi, of human crania with various degrees of dissection, specimens of human fetuses, whole preserved cadavers, and skeletons were found in this teaching museum. The lectures by Dr. Warren in Boston, dealing with human dissection, were secret. Being in charge of the Continental Hospital in Boston, Dr. Warren had relative ease in obtaining human bodies for dissection without usually resorting to taking bodies from the burying-ground. Warren also obtained at least four recently executed criminals for dissection.[51] One of his specimens, however, an old fat spinster, was more problematic. He had arranged with a cemetery caretaker to obtain this lady's body during the night after the funeral. Unfortunately, the absent-minded caretaker left the shovel next to the grave, which was promptly noticed the following day by relatives of the deceased. The discovery of this crime resulted in a request for a search warrant for the body from the Governor, who also being a member of the Harvard Corporation, refused to issue a warrant! This incident, though, was atypical for the new medical school in Boston in view of Warren's access to legitimate cadavers. In medical schools in other cities and towns, however, the shortage of cadavers often resulted in grave robberies at night, a condition which hardly helped the status of medicine in the minds of a public already dubious. Dissections were accordingly carried out in cellars and other secret places, and the public opposition to the practice of exhumation resulted in legislation against this practice. One such act was the law tendered in Connecticut in 1824 which prohibited the dissection of a body without the consent of relatives, subject to a large fine of $200–$2,000 or 1–10 years in prison. Further, according to this law public inspection of medical premises dealing with anatomy was authorized, as was the use of bodies of state prisoners without relatives. Elisha North, a foremost Connecticut physician (1771–1834), protested such a law, claiming that grave robbing was not really a theft; the remains were not owned by anyone, for the "owners" had relinquished all claims, and the body was no longer property useful to anyone, nor transferable from person-to-person.[37] Because of this chronic shortage of human cadavers for dissection, horses or other large animals were sometimes used, and a number of cases were recorded of outright murder of town drunks, whores, or "accelerated" deaths of the infirm by profit-making individuals who had contact with eager but naive professors of anatomy. In our "enlightened" time of the late twentieth century one at least has confidence in the legitimate procurement of human cadavers, and even increasing legislation is forthcoming on use and transfer of parts and various tissues in modern medicine— however, the problem of shortages has not been completely solved due to the large number of medical schools. The present writer recalls both the chronic shortage of cadavers at his previous Canadian medical school, not to mention his own American class in human dissection when all cadavers were headless — the heads having been shipped to some dental school — thus sparing the author from the laborious head and neck dissection!

Table 13
Notable Events in American Medicine, 1800–1825

1800	Benjamin Waterhouse introduced Jennerian vaccination in New England.
1801	Dr. David Ramsay published Progresses in XVIIIth Century Medicine, Charleston.
1802	United States Marine Hospitals at Norfolk (Virginia) and Boston (Massachusetts).
1802	Samuel Brown vaccinated 500 people in Lexington, Kentucky.
1803–8	Lewis and Clark explored the Rocky Mountains and sources of the Mississippi; they carried along smallpox vaccine.
1804	Philadelphia Medical Museum (a journal) started.
1804	Philadelphia Medical and Physical Journal started.
1805–26	First Boston Medical Library.
1807	College of Physicians and Surgeons (New York) founded.
1807	College of Medicine, University of Maryland (Baltimore) founded.
1808	Dr. David Hosack performed first ligation of femoral artery for aneurysm in America.
1809	Dr. Ephriam McDowell successfully performed oophorotomy in Danville, Kentucky.
1809	Dr. John C. Warren published *Cases of Organic Diseases of the Heart*.
1809	Yale Medical School founded.
1810	Dr. Daniel Drake published *The Climate and Diseases of Cincinnati*.
1811	Massachusetts General Hospital (Boston) established.
1811–14	Dr. Caspar Wistar published *System of Anatomy*, first U.S. systematic treatise on anatomy.
1812	The New England Journal of Medicine and Surgery and the Collateral Branches of Science started.
1812	Academy of Natural Sciences founded at Philadelphia.
1812	Bellevue Hospital (New York) established.
1812	Dr. Benjamin Rush published first American book on psychiatry.
1816	*Medical Sketches of the Campaigns of 1812, 13, 14* published by J. Mann in Massachusetts.
1817	Medical Society of the District of Columbia (Washington) founded.
1817	Quine Medical Library, Chicago, founded.
1818	Dr. Valentine performs ligation of innominate artery.
1818	Joseph Lovell was first Army physician to be appointed Surgeon General.
1819	Library, Harvard Medical School (Boston) founded.
1819	Medical College of Ohio founded.
1820	Cincinnati Commercial Hospital founded.
1820	Philadelphia Journal of Medical and Physical Sciences started.
1820	Philadelphia College of Apothecaries opened.
1821	Philadelphia College of Pharmacy founded.
1822	Samuel Thomson published *New Guide to Health* on use of botanical drugs.
1822	William Beaumont, M.D. acquired patient, Alexis St. Martin for gastric physiologic experiments.
1824	Academy of Medicine (Cleveland, Ohio) founded.
1824	Franklin Institute (Philadelphia) founded.
1825	University of Virginia (Charlottesville) founded.
1825	Jefferson Medical College established at Philadelphia.
1825	Fever hospital in New York City.
1825	*American Medical Biography* 2 vols. published by J. Thacher in Boston.

Chapter VII

Obstetrical Practice,
Midwifery and Accouchers

General Philosophy

The practice of midwifery during the early nineteenth century was well entrenched in Western Europe and the British Isles, but the relationship of this art to the general health care delivery system for the society, to the question of supervised training of the rather large numbers of midwives required, and to the question of professional rivalry between male physicians and female midwives was not dissimilar to problems which still exist in the twentieth century.

Paradoxically, although a Chair of Midwifery had been established in Edinburgh as early as 1726 and most centers of medical training in Western Europe, England and Scotland and the new United States had founded such posts by 1825, obstetrical surgeons were frequently downgraded by their fellow surgeons and physicians. Public acceptance of male midwives was not universally found, physicians argued amongst themselves over the alleged value of midwives for the natural phenomenon of normal, child delivery, and there existed the familiar pattern of a male obstetrician for the rich and a female midwife for the poor. It was felt by many that "to suppose an inadequacy in Nature to accomplish every requisite respecting the birth of the human species, is to imagine that chance, and not consummate wisdom, is concerned in this most important event."[1] In fact, male obstetricians themselves were a late addition to the medical world, coming into existence only during the seventeenth and eighteenth centuries. These male obstetricians formalized training programs for midwives, most particularly in France, such as at the Hôtel Dieu in Paris. In Britain the Society of Apothecaries attempted to persuade Parliament to authorize the examination and licensure of midwives in 1813, but this scheme failed, probably due to the Victorian taboos against teaching and discussion of the facts of life. Nonetheless, by this time considerable practical experience in midwifery was being recorded in the medical literature. One report, unique in that it referred to the remarkable success of a female midwife writing to the Manchester Lying-in Hospital, attests to a Sarah Roddry's having delivered over 5,000 babies, including 63 sets of twins, between 1817 and 1840, and never lost a mother! Dr. John Ramsbotham, who was lecturer on midwifery at the London Hospital and a male midwife or "physician-accoucheur" at the Lying-in Charity, stated that more than five thousand poor females delivered through his Charity annually, providing ample opportunities for observation of problematic cases. He further proclaimed[2] that

> The obstetric art has thus been brought to such a state of maturity, that little improvement can be expected, excepting from those who are engaged in the most extensive practice of it; and we are happy to find that they, whose office it is to assist the birth of mankind, and to relieve some of the miseries, and to avert some of the dangers, to which the fairer sex is exposed, are not less zealous in the cause of science than their brethern who have adorned the other branches of the profession by their exertions in our hospitals, fleets, and armies.

As a result *and* cause of the increased attention to the medical and surgical management of obstetrical problems in the early 1800's, and to the rising status of midwifery as a practice, a number of treaties on this subject were published, as illustrated by the following examples:

Practical Observations in Midwifery; with a Selection of Cases. Part 1. — by John Ramsbotham, M.D., London, 1821, 422 pp.

Essays on Various Subjects Connected with Midwifery. — by William P. Dewees, M.D., Carey and Lea, Philadelphia, 1823, 480 pp.

A Treatise on Midwifery; developing Principles which tend materially to lessen the sufferings of the Patient, and shorten the Duration of Labour. — by John Power, Accoucheur, London 1819, 270 pp.

Outlines of Midwifery, developing its Principles and Practice; with Twelve Lithographic Engravings. — by J.T. Conquest, M.D., London, 1820, 193 pp. and 1823, 224 pp.

The Principles of Midwifery; including the Diseases of Women and Children. — by John Burns (Fifth and Enlarged Edition) London, 1820, 519 pp.

Pratique des Accouchemens, ou Mémoires et Observations choisies sur les pointe les plus importans de l'Art. — by Madame La Chapelle. Paris, 1822.

Cours Pratique d'Accouchemens, avec une nouvelle Nomenclature des Présentations et Positions du Fetus, désignee sous le Nom générique de Pelvi Foetale. (Four Synoptical tables of maladies and treatments.) — by E. Moulin, M.D., Paris, 1821.

A Compendious System of Midwifery, chiefly designed to facilitate the Inquiries of those who may be pursuing this Branch of Study, illustrated by occasional Cases; with thirteen Engravings. — by W.P. Dewees, M.D., Philadelphia, Carey and Lea, 1824, 608 pp.

Archives de l'Art des Accouchemens, considers sous ses Rapports anatomique, physiologique, et pathologique. — Collected from the foreign literature by J.F. Schweighoeuser, M.D., Strasbourg, 1801, 187 pp.

Of course many other books on this subject were published during this period and the preceding century. A number of such monographs, particularly those appearing in the 1700's prior to the growth of "scientific" inquiry in the early 1800's, strongly protested the use of male midwives in this art,[3] primarily on pious grounds. These more sceptical books, proscribing male accouchers on a moralistic basis, had little influence as evident by the increasing use of male midwives. Stances on both sides of this issue continued to appear, however. One Dr. Kinglake, who saw no propriety in male midwives, contended that midwifery, as conducted by men in 1816, ought to be abandoned "as a busy, intermeddling, mischievous craft."[3] His opponent, Dr. Samuel Merriman, also of London, replied that accoucheurs are now (1816) preferred to the midwives

> because they have been proved to possess greater skill, greater judgment, greater mildness, greater patience, and greater decorum, and if men were very deficient in any one of these qualifications, it cannot be believed that they would be employed by the generality of females.[3]

Another accoucher, Dr. Joseph Adams expressed his view in the London Medical and Physical Journal (1816) that "every reader must be aware of two grand qualifications which, unless we could alter the race, must forever remain deficient in the female ... courage and corporeal strength."[23]

The published arguments in 1816 between Drs. Kinglake and Merriman over the advantages of female versus male midwives, respectively, are of interest since they provide some limited statistical data on the obstetrical risks recorded in lying-in hospitals of the day. One table,[3] drawn up by Dr. Bland, physician-man-midwife to the Westminister General Dispensary in London, delineates the observed complications of 1,897 cases of labor attended by midwives. There were reportedly:

68 women with wrong presentations of children

12 lingering labours requiring instruments

2 convulsions

9 haemorrhage, of which 3 died

5 puerperal fever

2 puerperal mania

1 supporation of the vagina and bladder

1 laceration of the perinaeum

5 oedema lacteum

thus, indicating that one in 18 cases had laborious or unnatural births and that one in 44 was attended with particular danger. Further data[3] of deliveries managed by midwives from other hospitals in France indicated that in 12,751 patients delivered in the Hospice de la Maternité in Paris (data published in 1812), 109 were cases of the child's head in the wrong position, and 394 of the child presenting preternaturally, i.e., an unfavorable presentation occurred once in every 26 labors. Statistics from the Maison d'Accouchemens in Paris, collected between 1799 and 1809, indicated that of 17,308 women delivered there, one of 26 deliveries had unfavorable presentations and one of every 25 women died at time of delivery. These data were used as arguments attesting to the need for the use of skilled male midwives or male obstetricians, rather than the traditional female midwife. It is of interest to note that this controversy exists to a degree even today, and usually hinges upon the requirements for highly skilled physicians/surgeons in problematic cases. Indeed, in Britain the training and regulation of midwives is constantly being revised, from the establishment of a Midwives Institute (1881), passing of various Midwives Acts (1902, 1936), lengthening of midwife training periods (3–6 mo. in 1917, single 47 week period in 1971), and various other changes.[4] In the early 1800's there was some discrepancy in the training and regulation of midwives in various Western European countries. It was contended in 1801 in the London Medical Review[5] that, though many valuable discoveries were made in the art of midwifery in France, there was a remarkable lack of proper regulations in the practice of midwifery. This conclusion was drawn by Dr. Jaques Frederic Schweighoeuser of Strasbourg, who further contended that German accoucheurs have long directed their united attention to both the advancement of the art and "to a severe vigilance over the conduct and ability of those who exercise the profession." While an element of truth exists in Schweighoeuser's statement, it also is biased by the rivalry known to exist between western European countries and the British Isles with respect to medical progress. Dr. Schweighoeuser, a strong advocate of the obstetrical arts, also concluded that it was only during the period 1700–1800, that the "art of midwifery, though highly important in itself, has been raised to the rank of science."[5]

Further examples of the controversy between human intervention and management of problematic deliveries, versus allowing the delivery process to take its own course without the use of *trained accoucheurs*, are noteworthy since this issue clearly depicts the emergence of scientific inquiry occurring during the early nineteenth century. A quotation by Atkinson, published originally in 1816[1] is illustrative:

> Of the supreme excellence, oeconomy, and beauty of Nature, he will be the most thoroughly convinced who examines her the closest; nevertheless it cannot be denied, that her operations would often be incomplete if left solely to the influence of the immediate causes that govern them. For this purpose the human intellect is often necessarily brought in aid, as in the cultivation of the ground, the removing weeds or excrescences which would otherwise prevent or retard fructification; and in destroying noxious animals which would annoy the senses, or interrupt the well-being of the more important orders of organized beings; also, in the prevention of diseases, no one will dispute the advantages of vaccination; and, I think, it is easy to prove, that in no instance is the judicious interference of art more necessary than in alleviating the distresses or averting the dangers incident to human parturition.

Another more tempered view on the general interference of man on parturitive functions was expressed in a review of Dr. John Power's 1819 treatise on midwifery:

> But it is not in parturition alone that the great power of Nature is cognizable; and there is strong reason to believe that the apparent perfection of her operations has sometimes led us to a devotion that has blinded us to her defects; her occasional incapacities; nay her irregular and even insalutary aberrations. Nor do we accuse *her* of these imperfections. We first desert Nature's standards; then turn a deaf ear to her calls, or run counter to her laws; and lastly, when we come to suffer the penalty of our follies, we expect that from Nature which we have not left her the power to perform.[7]

It was concluded by some[1,9,11] that an accoucher's attendance was a necessity in all cases of midwifery, since a *medical man* could watch and appraise any event requiring assistance such as hemorrhage, suppression or urine and preternatural presentation, etc., which are more easily remedied at the beginning than after a lapse of time. Further description of such obstetrical problems demanding employment of a "well-educated man" as midwife includes[1,6]

1) Laceration of the perineum
2) Exhaustion of the strength, by undue stimulants or frightful tales.
3) Convulsions
4) Uterine hemmorrhage
5) Danger to the child, by suffering the funis to remain tight about its neck.
6) Soothing the patient's mind, proper regulation of her diet.

Further, in reply to one of the opponents of the accoucher movement, who termed as "murder" the intervention of male midwives in fatal deliveries, Dr. Wayte of Calne replied[8]:

> If a hue and cry about "murder" and other intemperate nonsense are to restrain the just liberty of remarking on principles and practice in any department of the medical profession, there would be an end put to all independent and conscientious investigation; — the tyranny of opinion and adoption would usurp the place of discussion and correction; and erroneous prejudices would have a chance of being sanctioned, if not by "craft," at least by clamour and groundless opposition.

How reminiscent this is of the twentieth century conflict between antiabortionists and proponents of the discriminant use of abortion, the cry of "murder" by extremist, antiabortionist groups, and the scientific inquiry of causes and prevention of early, fetal malformations!

Physiologic Considerations

As with many physiologic concepts of the early nineteenth century, views of mechanisms of conception, uterine function, placental circulation, and delivery possessed elements of truth, as well as misconceptions which were nonetheless derived in a logical manner. Conception in the human, or the *theory of generation*, had been described by various continental physicians, including Gärtner of Copenhagen, and by the American, Dewees, who published midwifery treatises in Philadelphia.[9,10] It was generally accepted that the presence of semen at the ovaries was absolutely necessary for impregnation. It was believed that an absorption of "semen masculinum" from the internal surface of the vagina occurred, a phenomenon presumed to be aided by the rugose surface of the vagina, and that the semen was conveyed by "particular vessels" to the ovaries. It was presumed that seminal absorption could also take place at the labia, since conception was observed to occur when semen were applied only at that site. It was further alleged that the functions of the vaginal rugae were to 1) retain the semen so that it could liquefy there, 2) increase the area of the vaginal surface for seminal absorption, and 3) perhaps increase the degree of venereal pleasure. The latter function was questioned, however, since it was pointed out by Dewees[10] in 1823 that the doe (according to Harvey) had vaginal rugae in abundance yet only took the male "with reluctance and seeming pain," and that, "moreover, we see immodest women enjoying the veneral congress, when their vaginae, from their long continuance of their debililating habits, have the rugae destroyed." Thus, these early physicians seemed to miss the point that the vaginal rugae were merely a morphologic manifestation of folding of a collapsed tube, which can be observed also, particularly well in cross sectional views, in the esophagus.

It was questioned by Dewees why the vagina did "not also absorb the matter of gonorrhoea or lues," with consequent destruction of the ovaries, since it was presumed that there was a particular set of vessels within the vagina for seminal absorption. The explanation for the lack of vaginal absorption of the gonorrheal principle was that the particular set of absorption vessels were only "roused to absorption by their own particular stimulus, namely, the male semen."[10] Analogies to this alleged phenomenon were presented, as observed in the animal system; e.g., "light admitted to the tongue produces no sensation; yet let fall upon the eye, powerfully effects it," and "vibration of a musical chord or the tones of a flute, induce no change on the eye; but the ear is instantly influenced by them," and the intestinal lacteals selectively absorbed only the chyle, other portions of food not being a proper stimulus.

A suitable explanation for ectopic pregnancy, or "superfoetation," as it was termed in the early nineteenth century, had not yet been found to the satisfaction of the practicing midwives, although ectopic pregnancies were[12] reported. The birth of twins, of course commonly observed, was occasionally reported when problematic presentations occurred, such as interlocking heads.[13] The concept of impregnation, with respect to twins was that should there be but one ovum fit for the male influence, we shall have but one foetus, if two, we shall have twins, and so on. But for the most part there is only one; nature kindly providing against the neglect that must necessarily arise from several being produced at birth.[10]

The human menstrual cycle, and its relation to impregnation or multiple impregnatations was in part correctly interpreted. In this respect, the logic of the physicians in the early 1800's was based upon gross observations of time sequences, beliefs in the principles of animal economy regulated by nature, and theoretic deductions (unsupported by ample microscopic evidence) which were remarkedly accurate. The following passage, first published in 1823, summarizes their interpretation:

It would appear in general also, that a regular period elapses between the perfecting of each ovum; and hence we see women bearing children at stated intervals: for instance, every thirteen or eighteen months; every two, three, four, five, six, or seven years. Two, three, or four ova may chance to ripen (if we may so term it) at the same time; or in other words, may be in a condition to receive successfully the male influence; then we shall have, as we observed before, a corresponding number of children.

This law of perfecting the ova, however, is not immutable; here may sometimes happen a considerable variation in the term, but when in a condition may receive the stimulus of the male semen, and this may happen during the residence of a foetus in utero; hence superfoetation. But the time which elapses, for the most part is pretty uniform; and it would appear necessary also, that the first ovum or ova should be displaced before others can be perfected. This is a wise regulation of nature; otherwise, women who have lived long single, or been a long time deprived of commerce with man, would be subject to serious inconvenience; they would be liable to a litter of children. This rule obtains in other animals besides man.

Let us suppose now, a foetus to be occupying the uterus; the woman to have a subsequent connection with her husband; the semen to be absorbed and to meet with another ovum capable of being influenced by it; what will be the consequence? The ovum will be impregnated, and the ordinary changes will take place in the ovarium; the ovum will escape into the fallopian tube, and through it pass to the uterus; here it will meet with a feeble resistance from the membranes which already line the uterus, and consequently cover the openings of the tube; this resistance will however be soon overcome; either by the ordinary efforts of the tube, or by the ovum resting unusually long, and beginning to develop, obliging the mouth of the tube to open, while it contracts with unusual violence behind, from the stimulus of distention, and thus forces it forward and displaces the slightly adhering membranes, and by this means will effect a lodgment in the uterus by the side of the other, where it will be as completely developed for the period of its stay, as though it had been placed there at the same instant with the other. It will have its own membranes, water, and placenta; having nothing in common with the other but its nidus.

The role of the uterus as a recepticle (Fig. 36) for the developing fetus (referred to as the "uterine tumour" by early nineteenth centuries physicians) and as a muscular organ for placental attachment was often discussed, but its

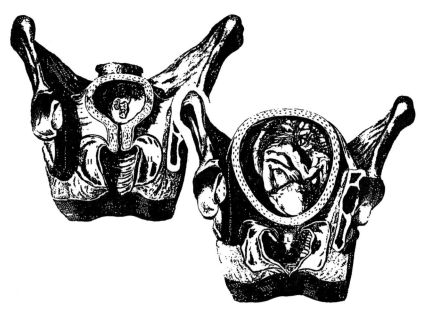

Fig. 36. Etching of early fetal development, as envisioned in the early nineteenth century. (Taken from 1792 text by W. Smellie[24])

nature somewhat disputed in the early 1800's. Notably, the uterus was said to contain both circular and longitudinal muscular fibers. Its tonic actions were known to be exerted in various degrees, including uniform strong contractions (e.g. during labor), feeble, nonproductive tonic contractions, and partial contractions involving only the fundus, the body, or the neck of the uterus. It was reasoned[9] that humans had lost much of their primitive, muscular strengths, hence providing one of the reasons women suffered during childbirth, but that the circular muscles of the uterus (as well as the heart and intestinal muscle) had retained their original vigor. In contrast it was believed that the longitudinal muscles of the uterus had lost their primitive vigor, were associated with uterine pain upon their contraction (e.g., after irritation of the uterus), unlike the circular muscular contractions which could produce "painless hour-glass contractions" of the uterus for hours. During the state of utero-gestation it was believed that a state of increased tonicity existed and was due to a "concentration of nervous energy round the uterine system."[7] It is to be noted that during the early nineteenth century the distinction had already been made, and the presently used terminology already adopted, between "voluntary" muscular contraction and control of skeletal muscle, "involuntary" contraction and control of the uterus, intestinal tract, heart, and the involuntary contractions (with optional voluntary control) of respiratory muscles.[14] From the foregoing comments it should not be concluded that uterine muscular activity was not disputed; indeed, Dr. Ramsbotham, a well-known lecturer on midwifery at the London Hospital, in his book in 1821 argued that the uterus was not, in fact, a muscular organ.[2] Although he contended that a fibrous texture could be discerned in the uterus upon dissection, its physiologic behaviour was not consistent with other muscles and it "ought not to be considered muscular."

Retroversion of the uterus, prolapse of the uterus, and cancer of this organ were often reported and well characterized by gross, anatomic descriptions in this period.[9]

An interesting physiologic concept concerning indirect effects of parturition was described by John Power, an accoucher, in 1819.[7] He conceived that a "metastatic translation of parturient energy" from the uterus to the heart and arterial system could occur in problematic cases causing feverish systems, or to the brain causing puerperal convulsions. He contended that this translation of parturient energy could be effected either by direct, or by "sympathetic excitement." An example of direct excitement was "spasmodic action of muscular fibres of the bladder," causing pain even at a time when uterine muscles were quiescent.

> Or it may happen that the irritation of the bladder, instead of producing increased actions of its own proper muscles, may excite sympathetic actions of a distant part, itself also remaining quiescent; there may be of the abdominal or other muscular parts ... producing sympathetic metastasis.

Such a condition allegedly could arrest labor. Dr. Power elaborated a philosophic and psychosomatic interpretation to this phenomenon, interestingly incriminating the whole of the social order:

> The predisposition to the metastatic state seems to depend upon an increased susceptibility of the system to be acted upon by associations or sympathies, excited by bodily or mental stimuli; which susceptibility appears to derive its origin from the present state of human society, as influenced by the acquisition of habits originally unnatural, and by the peculiarities of its moral education or constitution.[7]

He contended, however, that *predisposition* alone was not sufficient to give rise to metastatic actions, but that *local irritations* were essential, and might arise from uterine, vaginal, visceral, or mental irritations.

Selected Obstetrical Techniques, Drugs, etc.

Midwives of the early nineteenth century occasionally resorted to cesarean operations, sometimes with recovery of both mother and child. This was done as an abdominal cesarean (incision in direction of linea alba, above the pubis) or as a vaginal cesarean. The cesarean procedure itself had been used since the days of antiquity, being practiced on dead women, with the hopes of sparing infants, during the era of the first rulers of Rome, and being practiced on living women during the early sixteenth century. Several conditions were sanctioned as situations necessitating a cesarean during the nineteenth century.[15] One of these was the acute, accidental death of the mother, and physicians who neglected to attempt to save the infant is such cases were looked upon as criminals. As Dr. Michel stated in 1820, "What can be more horrid, than the burying of a living child within the entrails of a corpse!"[15] Such a crime in the time of the Romans was punished by death, and in 1749, Charles, King of the two Sicilies, ordered that any person hindering such type of cesarean operation should be arraigned as guilty of murder. It was recommended in the 1800's that accouchers be prepared to perform cesarean sections in any case of a pregnant woman near death.

A second condition in which the cesarean operation was recommended, in the early 1800's, was extreme narrowness of the female pelvis. There was in fact a divided opinion amongst accouchers as to whether or not cesarean operations should be performed on living mothers owing to the very high fatality rate for the mother. Nonetheless, it was accepted that a problematic, undelivered mother would succumb anyway, and attempts to save the child should be made. Indeed, records available to the early accouchers did show that some persons had survived several cesarean operations. The alternative procedure used by the midwives for cases of arrested deliveries due to extreme narrowness of the pelvis was the use of the crotchet, which required killing, mutilation, and piecemeal removal of the fetus. This latter method almost invariably resulted in death of the mother as well as the child.

Various other complications, such as exostosis (bony tumors) of the pelvis, extreme narrowness of the vagina, occlusion of the neck of the uterus by scarring or cancer, presence of steatomatous (fatty) tumors within the pelvic cavity, hernia (*irreducible hysterocele*) or rupture of the uterus, or extra uterine pregnancy had all been identified as conditions requiring cesarean operation.[15]

The use of forceps (Fig. 37) to facilitate delivery in difficult cases was employed and recommended by some of the accouchers of the early nineteenth century, though such practice remained somewhat controversial at this time. One Dr. Thomas Wales declared in 1818,

> Since I have been in practice, I have been called to many such instances, where midwives of very considerable experience have found it necessary to send for a male-accoucheur. The forceps in such cases, are generally applied without difficulty, and, in careful hands, always without injury to the mother and child.[11]

In the 1700's forceps had been used but more often misused, resulting in recommendations by various authorities in that century (Chapman, Gifford, Burton, Smellie) that they not be used at all. Prominent medical practitioners such as Professor Boer of Vienna, Dr. William Hunter, Madame Boivin (midwife to Hospice de la Maternité at Paris) discouraged used of the forceps. Dr. John

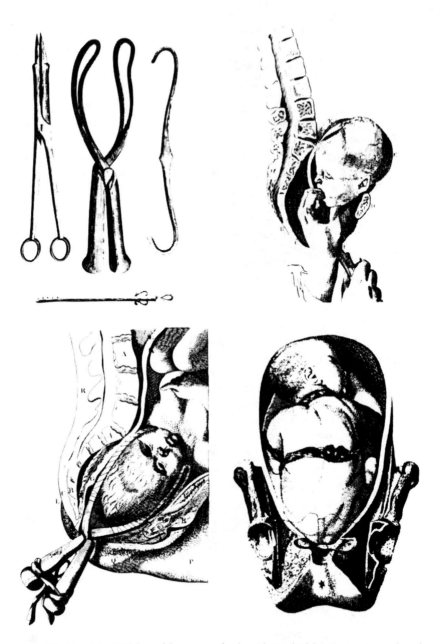

Fig. 37. Top left. Etching of forceps and other obstetrical instruments employed in the early nineteenth century. (Taken from 1792 text by W. Smellie[24])

Top right. Illustration of technique for using crotchet for delivery. (Taken from 1792 text by W. Smellie[24])

Bottom left. Cutaway diagram showing method for using forceps for delivery. (Taken from 1792 text by W. Smellie[24])

Bottom right. Illustration of fetal strangulation by umbilical cord, as envisioned in early nineteenth century. (Taken from 1792 text by W. Smellie[24])

Burns, Regius Professor of Surgery at the University of Glasgow, recommended restricted use of instrumental aids in delivery,[16] and a quotation from a review of his book on midwifery is instructive:

> It has fallen to our lot in various occasions to regret, that recourse to the forceps had not been more early sought. We have witnessed several instances in which the life of the child has been lost, for want of reasonable assistance from these instruments, and sometimes the mother has been placed in a very unwarrantable state of hazard from the delay. While therefore we join heart and hand with those who deprecate the hasty and intemperate use of instruments, we as earnestly insist upon the propriety of having timely recourse to them, when the circumstances of labour indicate a want of power in Nature, to discharge her duty satisfactorily.

The specific uses for the forceps have been outlined in 1820 by Dr. J.T. Conquest, Physician-Accoucheur to the City of London, in his book on midwifery.[17] He attested that the long forceps was a valuable instrument and most important substitute for the perforator and crotchet, which destroyed children. The instrument was to be used, 1) in cases of deformity at the brim of the pelvis and in which a little power beyond that of the uterus could expel the infant, and 2) in cases of hemorrhage, convulsions, etc., in which delivery was essential to the well being of the mother. Both long and short forceps were employed, with instructions for each type published.[17] Other authors[2,10] presented detailed criteria to be considered before instrumental assistance was used in delivery, criteria which ranged from the length of time the infant's head remained in the same situation in the pelvis, and the appearance of vaginal and uterine discharges, to the feelings of confidence or depression of the patient, or "the temperature of the weather at the time prevalent." One writer[10] suggested that "a rule for the time of applying the forceps has been formed from this circumstance; that, after the cessation of the pains, the head of the child should have rested six hours in such a situation as to allow the use of the forceps." However, a delay of this long of duration was criticized by most writers of this period.

A variety of drugs were used by midwives and male accouchers to alleviate the miseries of labor and to alter the time course of delivery. Opiates were employed in some cases of protracted labor. Dr. Ramsbotham[2] offered a judicious, philosophic comment on their recommended use in respect to labor pain:

> It appears to me that labour pains (properly so called) do form, and were intended by the greatest author of nature for the wisest purposes to form a constituent part of the act of childbirth; that they are inseparably attached to it as a cause; that they are merely an external evidence of the presence and progress of those powers by which the process is finally to be terminated, but without a due degree of activity in which, it must be pro-

> longed; and that they ought not generally speaking, or on application of a general principle, to be meddled with. I am certain they ought not to be entirely suspended: I have my doubts whether, except in very rare instances, any attempt should even be made to palliate them. Pain is certainly an evil and is universally depreciated as an evil; it seems always highly desirable to get rid of it as soon as we can; but labour-pain is established to bring about the happiest results.[17]

Although the use of very large doses of opium was recommended by some writers to restrain uterine hemorrhage, its indiscriminate use was condemned by Dr. Conquest,[17] physician-accoucher, who noted that it paralyzed "the contractile energies of the uterine and arterial fibres." He outlined its uses (at doses of 4–5 gr./2–3 hrs. intervals), which included uterine hemorrhage as a consequence of irregular contractions, and hemorrhage resulting in a loss of vital powers. Others, such as Dr. Ramsbotham[2] did not recommend repeated doses of opium for hemorrhage attributable to retained placenta.

Other pharmacologic agents were included in the *materia medica* of the nineteenth century accoucher. It was recognized that some of these might exert physiologic effects on the basis of suggestion, or a placebo effect. Notably, Dr. Samuel Akerly of New York[18] published a very wise statement of this phenomenon:

> In the present disposition of the medical world, we are apt to look upon quacks and empirical remedies with an eye of contempt. Many inert remedies are no doubt rendered efficient and powerful in the hands of these illegitimate sons of Esculapius, by the force of recommendation and the power they have over the miracle of their patients. Medicines are frequently given by them with a bold temerity unknown to the modest practitioner. Hence perhaps their frequent cures, which from their blaze conceal their failures.

Dr. Akerly advocated one agent, ergot, which exerted a real, non-placebo effect in inducing labor in difficult cases of parturition.[18] This agent was not in wide acceptance for use in Britain during the early 1800's although it had been an agent long known in Europe, and in the new United States by women as a home remedy for midwifery. It was known as *pulvis ad partum accelerandum*, and was obtained by pulverizing the seeds of rye which had been effected by a fungus in a moist environment. Ergot had been mentioned by Darwin as a disease to which grain was susceptible:

> Shield the young harvest from devouring blight,
> The smut's dark poison, and the mildew white;
> Deep-rooted mould, and ergots horn uncouth,
> And break the canker's desolating tooth.
> —Darwin, *Botanic Garden* Canto 4, line 541

In man, toxic effects of ergot had been mentioned as "mortification of extremities"[18] and Dr. Saillant had described that "Recherches sur la maladie convulsive epidemique attribué par quelques observateurs à l'ergot, et confondue avec la gragrene seche de Solognots."[19] However, its use in parturition had not been well documented and Dr. Akerly, in addition to calling attention to its use in difficult labor, also attested to its use for amenorrhea. Other agents employed by accouchers included pills containing gum aloe or other alkaline medicines (including milk) for the heartburn of pregnancy,[9] "internal antispasmodics" such as ether, ammonia, wine, camphor, and opium for the "sympathetic irritations" or muscular spasms attendant to pregnancy,[7] mild laxatives, such as "subacid fruit" to prevent constipation in patients recovering from post-partum, perineal lacerations,[20] laudanum (thirty drops) to induce uterine contractions in parturient cases,[6] and the volatile tincture of guaiacum for painful and obstructed menstruation.[10]

Other procedures were added to the repertoire of the midwife, such as the application of leeches[12] to the perineum for extra-uterine pregnancy (see also Chapter 3 on the Medicinal Leech), abdominal application of leeches for peritoneal inflammation attendant to postpartum, adherent placenta,[2] or blood-letting from the arm for prolonged delivery or retained placenta.[2]

Also, certain foods and life styles were proscribed or prescribed for a salubrious course of pregnancy or recovery from labor. Dr. John Clarke, Licentiate in Midwifery of the Royal College of Physicians, published an account[21] of the adverse effects of eating oysters after childbirth, and account which exemplifies the teaching of Broussais on human physiology. Dr. Clarke maintained that

> The state of pregnancy not only induces such a flow of blood to the head, as to dispose it to be violently affected by the strong exertions of labor, so as to induce puerperal convulsions; but also to render it liable to be particularly acted upon for some time after childbirth, by sympathy with the stomach, when indigestible substances, especially the fishes of the bivalve class (oysters) have been eaten.[21]

Others, such as Dr. John Barnes of Glasgow suggested in 1809 a rather more interesting recommendation for recovery from complications of delivery, "A removal to the country, and the use moderate exercise on horseback, will contribute greatly to the recovery!"[22]

Chapter VIII

Digestive Tract Disease and Gastrointestinal Physiology

Gastroenterologic Concepts Prior to 1800

By the close of the eighteenth century the gastrointestinal tract was an organ system that had assumed great importance. This was due not to a clear understanding that the medical practitioners had of this system, since they were extremely ignorant of the function and disorders of the alimentary tract, but because their holistic concepts of disease had adopted a centralized role for the gut. It should not be unexpected that diseases of nonviewable, internal organs, which are known today to be interdependent and regulated by complex neural and hormonal mechanisms, would be baffling to doctors at the end of the eighteenth century. These doctors could seldom rely upon surgical inspection of diseased or normally functioning human gut organs in this period of septic surgery without adequate anesthesia — patients would most often die after accidental or deliberate breach of the abdominal wall. Furthermore, the numerous autopsies examined during this period would usually reveal nonspecific morbid, or postmortem changes which, in the absence of an informed microscopic analysis, would contribute more to confusion than to pathophysiologic elucidation. The present author, who is a Professor of Gastrointestinal Physiology active in investigative endeavors pertaining to gastroenterologic disease, can readily sympathize with frustrations of medical diagnoses confronting physicians in the early nineteenth century. In spite of their admitted difficulty in treating disorders of the digestive system, doctors in this era placed a central importance on gut function vis-à-vis many diseases including even those remote from the abdomen. In part, this was attributable, particularly after 1800 in France, to the dogma of the esteemed physician, F.J.V. Broussais, who considered that many diseases resulted from peritoneal inflammation (to be treated by extensive blood-letting to remove excessive fluids causing the inflammation). Broussais felt that

> violent and long-continued corporeal exertions, violent and repeated contractions of the abdominal muscles in vomiting, the centripetal oscillations

of the blood in the cold stages of intermittents, and strictures of the colon
or rectum producing unnatural contortions and friction of the intestines on
one another,

caused peritoneal inflammation.[1] It can be correctly argued that beyond
France the specific teachings of Broussais would not have gathered great
momentum elsewhere in Europe and Britain during the earliest part of the
nineteenth century; however, the notion of vascular congestion and inflammation of the gut as a seat of fever and other symptoms was established prior to
Broussais, and was the rationale for the widely accepted practice of employing
blood-letting, drastic purgatives, glysters to the rectum, and blisters to the abdomen. These concepts, in existence before 1800, were summarized and propagated in numerous treatises published between 1800 and 1825 by Dr. Abercrombie of Edinburgh, Dr. Broussais of France, Dr. Gasc, Dr. Pemberton,
Dr. Montfalcon, and many others.[1] It should be noted that their use of the term
"peritonitis" differed from ours today. Theirs referred to either acute or chronic
"inflammations" which in fact covered everything from peptic ulcer, alimentary tract cancers, liver and biliary disease, etc., but current use is more
specific. "Peritonitis" today is a true inflammation of the peritoneum, frequently caused by perforation of the gastric or bowel wall or accidental opening of
the abdominal wall, and is ordinarily rapidly fatal unless treated by antibiotics
or physiologically confined by abdominal adhesions.

Dr. Fodera of Paris compared various medical doctrines of Broussais,
Rega, Prost, and others in 1821.[2] Prost outlined how no fever existed without
an accompanying inflammation of the alimentary canal. He described in his
work, "La medicine eclairée par l'observation et l'ouverture des corps," that the
gastric organ influenced, when diseased, other disorders, particularly in the
nervous system due to sympathies existing between these systems.[2] Today, in
modern western medicine we know the converse to be true, in that gastric function is significantly modulated by nervous and psychiatric factors. In modern
Russian medicine, which has a number of conceptual biases that are not accepted in Western Europe and North America, the central nervous system is
considered *the prime* regulator of most gastrointestinal functions or malfunc-
tions. Placing great emphasis on the central role of the digestive tract, Prost
had stated,

> The mucous membrane of the intestines has appeared to me to merit great
> attention, and I have constantly observed that of the organs of digestion
> with great care. This, though an extremely disgusting labour, will sooner
> or later, give a solid basis to medicine. It is difficult and almost impossible
> to describe with precision, the multitude of alterations that take place in
> these organs, which, however, correspond to the symptoms of the greater
> part of diseases. I have opened at least one hundred and fifty bodies of pa-
> tients, who died of ataxic fevers, without finding any thing peculiar in the
> brain; but have always seen inflammation of the mucous membrane of the
> intestines, either with or without erosions.

Undoubtedly, many of Prost's observations were postmortem changes, as bodies, chemically unpreserved, were frequently examined hours after death. After listing a number of specific axioms pertaining to irritation of the mucous membrane of the intestines and related diseases, Prost stated "that the disorders of these viscera have more influence on the brain, in proportion as their arterial system is developed, the red blood abundant, and the irritating cause active." He contended that

> The micro-gastric fevers, whether ataxic, adynamic or nervous, manifest themselves by the symptoms they occasion, 1st, by the different degrees of arterial development in the intestines, 2nd, by the nature of the alterations of the mucous membranes, 3rd, by the action of the bile, whether from its quantity or quality, 4th, by the production of worms, and the irritation they occasion,

etc.[2] Prost's writings had appeared before Dr. Broussais' well-known work, *Histoire des Phlegmasies ou inflammations chroniques*, 1st edition, Paris, 1808, and Broussais partially accepted the theories of Prost, with some reservations. Broussais also considered fevers to be of inflammatory nature and that the stomach or small intestine was the seat of these diseases, but he also believed that diseases had their organ-specific or determinate rather than general seats of organ.

In England in 1802, Dr. Edward Miller published concepts developed before 1800, including, "Some remarks on the importance of the stomach as a centre of association, a seat of morbid derangement, and a medium of the operation of remedies in malignant diseases."[3] He suggested that

> The importance of the stomach to animal life may be inferred from its being much more universally found in the structure of animals than the brain, heart and lungs, and from the deprivation of it being much more universally and speedily fatal than that of any or all of those vital viscera [a fact related to fatal hemorrhage from the ruptured stomach in the early 1800's, though we know today that totally gastrectomized patients can survive for many years]. In a state of health, the functions of the stomach, as the principal organ of assimilation, will give it a high rank among the parts of the system which support life. But it is in diseases that its principal powers and relations are unfolded to view. In fevers it is probably, in most instances, the first part affected, as it commonly affords the first notices of the approaching mischief. From its susceptibility of morbid action by noxious powers applied immediately to its surface, or to distant parts of the body with which it maintains sympathetic connection, it becomes not only the introducer of such action to the vital organs, but a centre of association, and as index of the most interesting circumstances concerning the accession, progress, remission, crisis and cure of diseases....[3]

Other writers, such as Dr. T. Sutton of London, published treatises on disease. His was titled "Considerations regarding Pulmonary Consumption," the term used for tuberculosis, rampant during the early nineteenth century. In this volume, Sutton noted that

> The first symptoms of disease in the case related, were in the bowels, and by degrees the disorder became a confirmed phthisis pulmonalis. Hence, through its progress, seeing every pulmonary symptom so mild, I was often led to suspect that *the emaciation and debility to be induced by some disease of the abdominal viscera....*[4]

Today, we know that tuberculosis can indeed be focused in the intestines, as well as the fact that the gastrointestinal tract can elicit a variety of nonspecific reaction to diseases which are centered anywhere in the body.

The digestive tract–central nervous system axis for disease was conceptually recognized in England as well as on the continent, as exemplified by the following quotation by Lespagnol in the Medico-Chirurgical Journal[5]:

> Our brethren in France are beginning to see the strong connection between the head and epigastric viscera, and their reciprocal influence exerted on each other, both in functional and structural diseases. The valuable writings of Cheyne, Abernethy, Curry, Yeates, and some other authors, however, seem to be little read or understood in France. The observations of M. Lespagnol are drawn principally from among children, where the gastro-cerebral sympathy is more evident than in those of a more adult age.

Furthermore, the editor of the *Medico-Chirurgical Review* said[6]: "But contagion produces also, directly or indirectly, a peculiar effect on the nervous system, which is chiefly evinced by the disturbed functions of the brain and of the stomach."

It is evident, therefore, from the foregoing paragraphs, that many early nineteenth century physicians placed an unrealistic and all-encompassing importance on the stomach with respect to overall disease manifestations. By the close of the eighteenth century acute abdominal disease had not advanced significantly since the time of Hippocrates and Galen,[7] but this was destined to change rapidly during the nineteenth century, largely as a result of experimentation, increasing and critical questioning of the old dogmas, and debate propagated by the increasing number of medical journals. By 1800, most acute abdominal diseases, which of course included a myriad of distinct organic and constitutional problems, were simply classified, according to Hippocratic precedent, as *colic*, if the pain was associated with recovery, or as *ileus*, if death was the prognosis, and this terminology was retained for several decades in the nineteenth century. By 1800, several distinct clinical entities within the range of acute abdominal diseases were recognized correctly, including strangulated hernia, and large bowel obstruction. As early as 1727, perforation of gastric ulcer had been noted by Christopher Rawlinson, and numerous cases of this disease had been described by the noted pathologist, Matthew Baillie, in his atlas of morbid anatomy published in 1799. Abercrombie's treatise on gastric diseases by 1828 had, as well, described two cases of duodenal ulcer. The first, and single, appendectomy had been performed by 1736 although the

In His Majesty's Ship Venerable, in 1814, 1815.—Crew, 600 Men

DISEASES.	May	June	July	August	Sept.	Oct.	Nov.	Dec.	Jan.	Feb.	March	April	May	June	July	Aug.	Ent. on Sick List	Died	Invalid.*	Cured
Continued Fever - -	6	4	3	6	0	4	4	2	2	1	0	11	13	3	6	3	68	1	4	63
Dysentery and Diarrhœa	1	6	2	9	3	6	2	4	2	1	5	10	3	5	6	7	72	3	2	67
Hepatitis, Splenitis, &c.	3	3	2	0	0	1	2	1	3	1	1	0	0	3	6	0	26	1	4	21
Phthisis Pulmonalis -	0	2	1	1	2	0	1	2	0	2	1	0	1	1	3	0	17	2	7	8
Pneumonia - - - -	0	0	0	0	0	1	0	0	0	0	0	0	0	2	0	0	3	2	0	1
Cholera - - - - -	0	1	0	1	0	0	0	0	0	0	0	1	1	0	0	0	4	0	0	4
Catarrh ⎫ †-	4	1	1	3	1	4	5	0	1	0	1	3	0	2	5	5	36	1	0	35
Rheumatism ⎭	2	0	1	4	2	2	2	2	1	0	1	5	5	2	2	0	31	0	0	31
Colica Pictonum - -	0	0	0	0	0	0	1	0	5	3	0	1	0	0	1	2	13	0	0	13
Erysipelas - - - -	1	2	0	2	0	1	0	0	1	2	1	1	1	0	0	0	12	1	0	11
Ophthalmia - - -	1	1	0	3	4	1	1	1	1	0	0	0	1	1	0	1	16	0	1	15
Hydrothorax - - -	0	0	0	0	0	0	1	0	0	0	0	0	0	0	0	0	1	1	0	0
Icterus - - - - -	0	0	0	0	1	0	0	0	0	0	0	0	0	0	0	0	1	0	0	1
Cutaneous Eruptions -	0	0	0	0	1	1	1	0	1	0	0	0	0	0	1	0	5	0	0	5
Maniaϯ - - - -	0	1	1	0	0	0	1	0	1	0	0	0	1	0	1	0	6	0	2	4
Fish Poison - - - -	0	0	0	3	3	1	0	0	0	0	0	0	0	0	0	0	7	0	0	7
Constipation - - -	1	0	0	0	0	0	0	0	0	0	0	0	0	0	0	0	1	0	0	1
Convulsions - - -	0	1	0	0	0	0	0	0	0	0	0	0	0	0	0	0	1	0	0	1
Psora - - - - -	2	0	0	0	0	0	0	0	0	0	0	0	0	0	0	0	2	0	0	2
Phlegmon - - - -	9	6	13	7	8	11	2	1	9	5	5	6	3	3	6	7	101	0	0	101
Otitis - - - - -	0	0	0	0	1	0	0	0	0	0	0	0	0	0	0	0	1	0	0	1
Nephralgia - - -	0	0	0	0	0	0	1	0	0	0	0	0	0	0	0	0	1	0	1	0
Nostalgia - - - -	0	0	0	0	0	0	1	0	0	0	0	0	0	0	0	0	1	0	1	0
Lues Venerea - - -	6	2	2	0	0	2	1	3	1	5	2	0	8	3	1	2	38	0	2	36
Anomalous - - - -	0	3	1	2	2	0	0	4	0	0	4	1	0	0	0	0	17	0	0	17
Ulcers - - - -	3	4	2	0	0	0	0	0	1	0	2	3	1	0	0	2	18	0	1	17
Wounds and Accidents	8	12	8	22	8	14	11	7	9	3	10	15	8	6	11	23	175	2	1	172
TOTAL -	47	49	37	63	36	49	37	27	38	23	33	57	46	31	49	52	674	14	26	634

* In this Column are included those Cases sent to England for cure, or sent there because supposed incurable.

† These were all well marked and acute cases.   ‡ This Column contains two relapses of the same case.

Fig. 38. Distribution of diseases and other health related problems on shipboard in 1814–1815. As expected this occupation was associated with numerous wounds and accidents. Dysentery and diarrhea were commonplace on the ship, as they were on land.

nature of acute appendicitis was not understood at that time. By 1812, however, acute inflammation localized to the appendix had been noted during postmortem analysis of a five-year old by James Parkinson, and two further cases of appendicitis were described in Paris by Louyer-Villermay in 1824.[7] Dysentery and diarrhea constituted, however, the majority of gastrointestinal complaints (Fig. 38).

Concepts of Normal, Gastrointestinal Physiology Prior to 1800

The beginnings of a true, in-depth understanding of the normal physiologic mechanisms of the gastrointestinal tract did not begin prior to the end of the nineteenth century, since this required a certain, minimal understanding of protein and enzyme chemistry. Even in modern times, it can be stated that, although considerable gastrointestinal physiology has been known even since the 1940's, the biochemical era of gastrointestinal physiology has just begun to take place during the past two decades, and a host of new gastrointestinal, polypeptide hormones have been identified and chemically characterized, but are still poorly understood from a physiologic standpoint. At the close of the eighteenth century, inorganic chemistry was also more advanced than physiology. The early concepts of digestion brought forth various hypotheses of "putrefaction," i.e., digestion as a result of heat generated by the stomach or consequent to mechanical activities of the gut, or "fermentation," which was vaguely defined by 1800, in contrast to its present-day specific chemical connotation. Table 14 outlines some of the historic landmarks and lesser contributions in gastrointestinal physiology which had been achieved prior to 1800. Thus, by the dawn of the nineteenth century, the physiologic concept of digestion was vague, such as that described by Albrecht Von Haller in his 1803 physiology monograph:

> ... into the stomach ... the ailments are let down ... as alkalescent flesh, rancescent fat, or acescent vegetables. Here they are digested in a heat equal to that of incubation, imparted by the contiguous heart, liver and spleen ... The aliments are macerated in a moist place with much air ... at the same time they begin to corrupt into a nauseous liquid, often acescent, but at other times putrescent.[8]

Table 14
Milestones or Lesser Contributions
in Gastrointestinal Physiology Achieved Prior to 1800

First Discovery of Intestinal Lacteals	Gasparo Aselli (1581-1626)
Analysis of Human Weight Changes After Eating	Santorio Santorio (1561-1636)
Early Speculations about Digestion	Franciscus de le Böe (Sylvius) (1614-1672) J.B. van Helmort (1577-1644)
Experimental Collection of Pancreatic Juice in the Dog in 1664	Regner de Graaf (1641-1673)
Description of Gastric Juice in the Buzzard (kite) and its Digestive Actions	René Antoine F. de Réaumur (1683-1757)
First in Vitro Proof of Digestive Power of Human and Animal Gastric Juice. Studied Actions of Saliva	Lazaro Spallanzani (1729-1799)
Early Reports on Fish and Bird Lymphatics	William Hewson (1739-1774)
Provided Foundation for Modern Views of Function of Lymphatics	William Cumberland Cruiskshank (1745-1800)
Early Studies of Human Diet, Gastric Juice, etc.	William Stark (1740-1770) Edward Stevens, M.D. Thesis in 1777 Charles Darwin I (1758-1778)

Characterization of Gastric Diseases, 1800–1825

As delineated above, gastric ulcer and mucosal vascular changes, particularly as interpreted postmortem, of the inner surface of the stomach were noted with interest during the early nineteenth century. In France, Vanderschilt[9] and Villeneuve[10] described gastric inflammation and Richond[11] associated the appearance of apoplexy as a sympathetic response to gastric disease, in Bordeaux. Human and animal autopsies performed in England also stressed the relationship between vascular changes of the gastric mucosa with inflammation, as described by Yelloly and others.[12] Of particular interest, however, was Yelloly's account in 1815, since in describing the vascular appearance of the stomach at postmortem dissection, he took scientific steps to quantify his observations, listing for 12 patients the weight in grains of the "villous coat" and of the combined "peritoneal and muscular coats" of his deceased patients.[11] Dr. Yelloly attempted to correlate the thickness of various regions of the stomach with its susceptibility to autodigestion by gastric juices, in relationship to the vascularity. Even today, in modern times, a "vascular component" to the etiology of peptic ulcer disease, and especially to stress ulceration of the human stomach, remains a topic of considerable interest.[13]

The vomiting of blood (melena) was reported with interest in a number of case histories.[14] We know today that this might appear as fresh, red blood, such as from a fresh, acute gastric ulcer bleed or from bleeding esophageal varices, but it may also be manifest as a black vomitus, representing blood altered by acidic gastric juice. Isaac Cathrall reported in 1800,[15] in what was described as a "pointed and sententious production" of 32 pages, the association of "black-vomit" with the last stage of yellow fever in Philadelphia. Dr. Cathrall chemically analyzed this black vomit and concluded that it contained "a considerable proportion of water, tinctured with resinous and mucilaginous substances, … (and) a predominant acid, which is neither the carbonic, phosphoric, or sulphuric." Cathrall did not identify the black material as blood; however, his description of the presence of acid, which was not one of the inorganic acids mentioned above, was a notable achievement, since it appeared prior to Prout's 1804 discovery of hydrochloric acid of gastric juice. Cathrall tested his black, gastric refluxed material on his own and his friend's lips and tongue, and in diets experimentally fed to cats, a dog, and two birds. He considered and rejected the possibility that it might be a mixture of blood and bile, and finally incorrectly concluded that it was "an altered secretion from the liver."

Penetration of the stomach by gastric ulceration or accidental or wartime wounding was often reported[16, 19] in the early nineteenth century in patients, and even in domestic animals afflicted with ulcer.[20] Usually death ensued, but in some cases adhesion of the peritoneal coat of the stomach (confined ulcer) and cicatrix formation was observed.[19] It is interesting to note that in this recent post–Napoleonic period, it was widely known that Napoleon suffered a gastric affliction. In England, a case history was reported in 1821, in respect to a patient with assumed gastric ulcer, that "the following case, bearing no tri-fling analogy to that of the once renowned, but how nearly forgotten, Napoleon Bonaparte."[21] If only that writer could observe how Napoleon is still remembered even today! The author of this case history noted that in this patient with stomach ulcer

> a variety of evacuant medicines were used, but gave him no relief (and) fomentations and anodyne embrocations procured only temporary benefit, ... and as all the ordinary remedies had failed in affording alleviation to his distress, he was advised to try the effect of sea-bathing.[21]

Gastric stricture was also identified as a clinical entity in 1816 by Shirley Palmer, M.D. It was classed as a primary or secondary disease; the former condition resulting from tumors, or ulceration, and secondarily to morbid conditions of the liver or pancreas which might cause stricture of the gastric organ.[22] Gastric cancer was noted in a number of reports in the early nineteenth century. Then, as now, it would have been an almost one hundred percent fatal disease with rapid progress from its early clinical symptomology to death of the patient. We know today that gastric cancer has significantly decreased in incidence, particularly in Western Europe and North America, during the past three decades.[23] Whether this suggests that its incidence was much higher in the early nineteenth century, is not known or indeed ascertainable, because of unreliable early records and inadequate diagnoses of early times. However, those types of occupations and lower socioeconomic classes which are today identifiable as *high risk* to stomach cancer,[23] would have been more prevalent in the early nineteenth century. In contrast, gastric cancer generally is seen in older age persons and is relatively rare below the age of 40 years, and a much lower percentage of the early nineteenth century population was over 50 years of age. There is a confusing point with respect to terminology of gastric cancer then and now. Presently, one specific type of gastric cancer is known to be diffusely distributed on the gastric surface and is termed "scir-rhus cancer"; this type is less prevalent than the more common "intestinalized type" of gastric cancer today. At the beginning of the nineteenth century, the term "scirrhus of the stomach" was used indiscriminately in reference to conditions that were benign peptic ulcer, or occasionally gastric cancer. The French workers, Bayle and Cayol, described[24] the symptomatology of scirrhus of the stomach in a manner which was very compatible with peptic ulcer disease, symptoms that persisted for years (which would have been unlikely for gastric carcinoma). They stated that on postmortem inspection, "the internal surface of the scirrhus or cancerous part is generally prominent and uneven, and it is here that the ulceration always begins." We know today that ulceration frequently occurs at the site of a gastric tumor, but most gastric cancers probably do not originate from a previously benign gastric ulcer.[23] The so-called scir-rhous condition of the stomach, cited in *The Surgeon's Vade Mecum* of 1813[27] and by many writers[26] of this period, was considered to be fatal: viz, "Scirrhus, once formed, forbids the adoption of a curative plan. The efforts of art should merely be to palliate symptoms, and to retard, as much as possible, the ulceration of the tumor."[27] Dr. Abercrombie described "this affection is, of course, beyond the reach of medicine,"[28] and Broussais described typical, rapidly fatal gastric cancer in a soldier.[29] Recommended therapy for ulcer or for the "inflammatory state of the mucous membrane" of the stomach varied. Dr. John Cheyne recommended in 1827, as initial therapy, the application of leeches, fomentations, blisters, and enemata,[30] and if that failed to reduce fever or fullness of the stomach, he used purgative medicines. For treatment of "excessive dilatation of the stomach, without any obstruction of the pylorus," Dr. Andral recommended "leeches applied to the epigastrium, and magnesia and various antispasmodics given in turn."[31] Dr. John Elliotson in 1820 employed "prussic (hydrocyanic) acid," given 2–5 minims ("one minim being nearly two drops") per day for dyspepsia, pain in the epigastrium, flatulence, vomiting, etc. This agent was derived from "laurel water," and its toxicity was tested in animals, to which it was sometimes lethal.[32] The antacid, "white oxide of bismuth" was found beneficial in 1820 by Dr. Yeats, Dr. Bardsley of Manchester, Dr. Marcet, and others for gastric pain. Magnesia and chalk in cinnamon water was also effective in reducing pain.[33] A number of these remedies were not novel to this era, but had been used since ancient times. The internal administration of ice was used for treating "irritability of the stomach" in 1821,[34] as well the driving of a gold or silver needle, into the stomach and holding it there for four or five minutes.[35] This later form of acupuncture was also claimed to cure convulsive cough in 1817; it was not a commonly used remedy in the early nineteenth century. Dr. Stone of London used mercury and unguentum hydrargyri fortius (of the London Pharmacopoeia), which consisted of equal parts of quick-silver (mercury) and lard, rubbed nightly on the epigastric region.[36] As described in Dewees' book on midwifery, published in Philadelphia (1823), alkaline medicines (with antacid properties) were recommended for heartburn caused by reflux of gastric contents into the esophagus.[37] In this same monograph, it was suggested that when alkaline antacids failed to overcome the acidity of the stomach, administration of other acids, such as lemon juice, was beneficial.[38] Diet therapy was also recommended for gastric pain; specifically, Dr. Dale recommended in 1817 "such food only as with difficulty passes into the acetous fermentation; animal food, with a small quantity of hard biscuit and water."[39]

Gastric surgery (Fig. 39) was occasionally resorted to in France, England and elsewhere during the early 1800's, sometimes (rarely) with success and recovery of the patient.[40] [41] Dr. Percy, a British surgeon, gave good advice about suturing gastric wounds of men receiving knife and sword wounds during the war. He advised[41] that the objective of the suture was not to unite immediately the lips of the wound in the gastric membranes, but to prevent the effusion of food, drink, blood, and pus into the abdominal cavity. Percy stated that "it may be proper to observe, that divided membranes do not heal themselves: it is by their adherence to the parts with which we hold them in

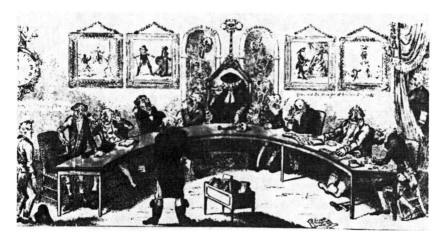

Fig. 39. Etching by Cruikshank, entitled "The Examination of a Young Surgeon" and completed in 1811. This illustration typified the widespread use of caricature in Great Britain during the early nineteenth century, and in this case satirized the Royal College of Surgeons. (Original on file at the National Library of Medicine, Bethesda, Maryland.)

contact that their wounds are cured." It was generally held at this time that stomach wounds are always fatal and should not be touched. Another excellent contribution by an early nineteenth century surgeon was that of Dr. Jukes, published 1823.[42] He described a suture tube which, when placed into the stomach via the oral route, could be used to withdraw poisons from the stomach. His device and technique was remarkably similar to the modern nasogastric tube used today for gastric analyses or gastric cooling. Jukes' tube was an

> elastic gum tube, a quarter of an inch in diameter, and two feet and a half in length, terminating at one extremity in a small globe of ivory, with several perforations; the other extremity is adapted, either by screw or by plug to an elastic bottle of sufficient size to contain at least a quart of liquid, and having a stop-cock fitted to it, in a similar manner as in the hydrocele bottle...

Jukes tried his device first on dogs and then on himself and others, including his assistant surgeon in Westminister, Mr. James Scott. His technique was as follows:[42]

> The patient ought to be placed on the left side, and the globulated end of the tube be then carefully passed to the greater curvature of the stomach, either through the mouth or nostril, as may be thought proper. Having previously filled the bottle or syringe with warm water, at the temperature of 150°, screw or plug it to the tube, turn the stop-cock, and gently force the contents into the stomach. The then diluted contents are to be im-

mediately withdrawn by pulling up the piston; or, if the bottle be applied, the same effect will ensue from its elasticity enabling it to recover its original form, by which the fluid contents will return, charged with the poison. This operation ought to be repeated, till the water, which is withdrawn, becomes clear and tasteless.

Diseases of the Liver and Biliary System, 1800–1825

We know today that the liver plays a central, or important secondary role in many diseases due to its complex biochemical and detoxification mechanisms which affect a wide variety of bodily functions. However, in the early nineteenth century, its functions were obscure, and physicians were able only to report on its variable, morbid appearances upon gross inspection at autopsy, and to speculate upon its role in production of bile. Matthew Baillie, M.D., (1761–1823), Physician Extraordinary to the King of England, presented in 1783 for the first time in any language, a pathology textbook entitled, *The Morbid Anatomy in Some of the Most Important Parts of the Human Body*,[40] which was the first systematic and codified pathology text. Dr. Baillie had studied under his famous uncle, the outstanding anatomist, William Hunter, who was brother to the well-known surgeon, John Hunter. Baillie's textbook presented morphological descriptions of various liver diseases, which fell into categories of "common tubercle of the liver," "large white tubercle of the liver," "soft brown tubercles of the liver," "scrofulous tubercles of the liver," "liver flaccid, with reddish tumours," "liver very soft in its substances," "liver very hard in its substance," and "hydatids of the liver." Although Dr. Baillie presented detailed and colorful verbal descriptions of these hepatic morphologic changes, it would be hazardous to attempt to identify each of his pathological entities with specific liver diseases as known today. Most of his entities, however, probably corresponded to different stages of cirrhosis or tuberculosis infiltrating the liver. Baillie did associate increased "common tubercles" of the liver with "hard drinkers, male sex, and older age."

Enlarged liver and jaundice, of course, were commonly noted, as well as gallstone disease. Powell described, in 1821[41] how:

Whenever violent pain takes place in the epigastric region of the abdomen, exacerbating in paroxysms accompanied by sickness, yellowness of the eyes and skin, and urine, by clay-coloured faeces, and without any proportionate increase of action in the circulation, biliary concretions are supposed to be forcing through the ducts; and when these symptoms abate, it is inferred that their passage into the duodenum has been effected.

This physician searched for the passed gallstone in fecal material collected from such patients. He noted that most such patients were females, as today we note that gallstone disease is most prevalent in overweight middle-aged females. Dr. Powell reported that a sedentary life contributed to the risk of being affected with gallstones. He also recorded how he believed psychic factors elicited jaundice, and biliary tract malfunction:

> The passions have a most remarkable effect on the secretion, and also on the ducts of the liver. A fit of anger will so derange the state of bile, as to tinge the skin yellow in a few hours. A sudden and unnatural acrimony of a secretion may very readily excite the organic contractibility of a tissue composing a canal, and thus occasion a stricture of its calibre for the time being. In this way, I have no doubt that jaundice is often induced by mental emotions, as anger, jealousy, grief, etc...[41]

Therapy for biliary tract obstruction, as recommended by Dr. Powell, consisted of treating patients in a state of acute paroxysm with a warm bath, warm fomentations, blood letting by leeches, and blisters. Also, he would administer, internally, "pretty large does of opium and hyoscyamus, and then acting on the bowels pretty briskly by compound extract of colocynth, calomel, and hyoscyamus, aided by purgative enemata to solicit the peristaltic action."[41] Some two decades earlier in his career, Dr. Powell had hypothesized that "the difference between biliary concretions (gallstones) and bile depends merely upon the relatively increased proportion of oxygen in the latter."[42] Observations on his chemical experiments with gallstones led him to believe that bile contained a peculiar resin, rendered soluble in water by its union with soda. He was almost correct in this analogy; we know today that bile has detergent properties, and its solubility in water is attributable to the polar groups residing on one side of the bile acid molecule, the other side being more soluble in lipid.

Mercury was also recommended in the treatment of "schirrous liver," and was used as a purgative, with supposed beneficial actions on impaired function of the "ductus communis choledochus."[36]

Liver disease was characterized as acute or chronic, with

> a congestive state of the vena portarum and its branches in both forms of the complaint; but in the acute one, there is a higher degree of this congestive state, giving rise in its turn, to a certain degree of venous congestion in those organs of the abdomen whose circulation is associated with that of the liver.[43]

Today, we would, with some modification, state the converse, as the more severe and chronic forms of "congested" liver are attended with an increase in portal venous pressure, and subsequent varices in the more distant but associated blood vessels.

A complete treatise[44] on diseases of the liver was published by Dr. William Saunders; sales of the first two volumes being so great that volume three was published in London in 1803. This concise and well-written monograph was one of the most scientific and outstanding medical books of this era, and Saunders candidly stated the limits of current knowledge of the hepato-biliary system.

Diseases of the Intestines, 1800–1825

In 1800–1825 maladies of the intestines, then as now, constituted a large percentage of patient complaints and difficult diagnoses. Intestinal problems were frequently associated with fatal outcomes since surgery and adequate treatment of severe diarrhea were not feasible at this early date. Dysentery, obstructed and strangulated bowel, and cancers of the lower digestive tract were commonly observed at the turn of the eighteenth century.

The surgeon, Dr. John Howship, published in 1820 a 176 page monograph on diseases of the lower intestine, the verbose title of which covered half a page. His work, reviewed by the editor of the Medico-Chirurgical Review,[45] elicited the following noteworthy point:

> The establishment of dispensaries is a measure that must tend to give an amazing impulse to the progress of medical and surgical science. In these institutions, diseases are seen earlier among the poor than they otherwise would; and as the medical officers, in general, are young, zealous, and not distracted by the multifarious exertions of extensive private practice, they study the phenomena of diseases more carefully, record them more accurately, and communicate them more freely, than before these eleemosynary mansions were erected. These advantages are certainly not without some alloy, as it respects medical literature. The just balance between facts and deductions; that is, between cases and principles, is somewhat deranged, and the press pours forth the former in such a torrent as threatens a deluge rather than fertilizing irrigation. Nevertheless, as individual cases form the basis of medical science, in the same manner as grains of sand form the mountain, and drops of water the ocean, we must not object to this multiplication, in this infantile period of our knowledge.[45]

Dr. Howship described cases of "ulceration of the internal surface of the intestines" which may have been what we know today as ulcerative colitis, but this is not verifiable, inasmuch as there are a number of causes of lower bowel ulceration. Prolapsed ani, hemorrhoids, anal fissures, and rectal tumors were also described in Howship's monograph.[45] Exercise was recommended as a therapy, especially for constipation in the elderly and for those in the "sedentary classes." Increasing the function of the skin (enhanced sweating) was also described as beneficial for constipation, and bathing in warm mineral water was recommended to enhance skin function. Others, such as Calvert, thought that food (via what we now know as the normal, gastro-colic reflex) could contribute to the production of hemorrhoids, as he indicated

> that the excitement of the stomach is sympathetically communicated to the colon and rectum is proved by the almost immediate effect of breakfast in producing an action in the bowels, in a state of good health. So the morbid excitement of the same organ by stimulating food and drink, produces a tendency to haemorrhoids through the same medium.[46]

The duodenum (proximal small intestine) was considered by Yeats[47] to be the seat of a variety of ailments, including:

> The appetite declines, or becomes capricious; flatulence is troublesome; languor and lassitude are considerable, accompanied by sense of weakness in the lower extremities, occasional chills, feverish heats, pain and sense of weight in the right hypochondrium and across the loins, torpid bowels with dark coloured faeces passed without being figured; urine of a mahogany colour, sometimes transparent, sometimes with a lateritious or white sediment, or thick like gruel and water; slight nausea, restless nights; white crusted tongue, brown towards the roots; occasional giddiness or headache, or affection of vision; pulse little accelerated, ... despondency, and, after some time, a yellow tinge in the eye ...

Happily, we can say today that, aside from common duodenal ulcer, there are relatively few maladies of the duodenum, and that most all of Yeats' claims are untrue.

Flatus, or gastrointestinal gas, and its abdominal sounds, borborygmi, were noted as important physiologic findings with clinical significance related to obstructive bowel disease.[48] Its origin from ingested food or endogenous formation, and its composition were discussed. It was said to consist of "carbonic acid, and carburetted or sulphuretted hydrogen."

Ileus, described earlier in this chapter as a general term for serious, often fatal maladies of the intestinal tract, was thought by Dr. John Abercrombie to result from an "inverted motion or action of the intestinal tract."[49] In references to Morgagni, Abercrombie cited his own observations of reverse peristalsis, and the vomiting of glysters, or suppositories that had been administered per rectally. Thus, obstruction was ruled out as a cause of ileus. Ileus was treated by warm bath, opiate glysters, blisters to the abdomen, and blood-letting. Obstruction of the bowels was known for its dire consequences, as a strangulation of the small intestines with ensuing gangrene and death.[50-53] Treatments for obstruction varied from administration of castor oil, salts, rhubarb, calomel, Epsom salts, oil of turpentine, olive oil, barley water, blood-letting, glysters, and quicksilver. Surgery was seldom resorted to; the writer Monfalcon in 1818 pondered:

> But he hesitates not to prefer the efforts of Nature to the interference of Art. Who will believe that the persons who have recovered, after the discharge of a great length of gangrenous intestine by the anus, would have done equally well under the attempts of a surgeon to destroy the volvulus by the operation of a gastrotomy?[54]

Obstruction of the colon by large, endogenously-formed stones,[55] laceration of the ileum by a kick from a horse,[56] ulceration, appearing most frequently[57] in the lower ileum (Crohn's disease?) but also in the colon,[58] and perforation of the bowel by parasites or disease[59,60] were also discussed in the literature.

Chronic diarrhea was also a problem of the intestinal tract, as discussed in letters to Dr. Benjamin Rush from Dr. Hayes of Maryland (1801), in England, and elsewhere.[61,62] It was treated, similarly to obstruction, by cupping glasses applied to the abdomen in obstinate cases,[63] by saline, calomel, mercurial, or ipecacuan purgatives.[63,64] The table in Figure 38 presents a listing, compiled in 1816 and published in 1818, of all diseases presenting for a two-year period on His Majesty's Ship Venerable. It is evident that, in addition to the expected high risk to sailors of wounds and accidents, a phenomenon that remains constant even today, that dysentery and diarrhea constituted a significant percentage of all disorders observed. This was true on land as well as at sea, and infant mortality during 1800–1825 was enhanced greatly by uncontrolled, severe diarrhea due to multiple causes.

Normal Gastrointestinal Physiology, 1800–1825

To begin an account of the physiologic status of the gastrointestinal tract of the early nineteenth century, it is useful to reiterate the words of the time. For example, the famous physiologist Majendie had said that, "Physiology, or the science which aims at elucidating the powers and functions of the animal body is emphatically in its infancy."[65] An editor of *The Lancet* had stated in 1825[66] that

> so little indeed are the anatomy and appearances of the mucous membrane of the alimentary canal studied in this country (England), that we feel no hesitation in saying that nine surgeons out of ten cannot tell a healthy from a diseased portion when it is shown them.

It was agreed, however, that

> the affections of the stomach, liver, and digestive organs in general, have always been a prolific source of medical writings; probably because the subject is a popular one, and comes home to men's feelings, as interfering with their every-day enjoyment.[36]

Aside from the philosophic comments on the status of physiology, occasional nonscientific biases found their expression in the early nineteenth century medical literature such as the following comment by an English editor, indicating some international animosity:

> If Dr. Wilson Philip had been as well skilled in puffing as he is in experimenting, he would, we are persuaded, have acquired a much higher reputation, than his modesty and plain good sense have been able to procure for his originality of research in medicine and physiology. His character is, in this respect, truly English, without a particle of the forwardness and frippery, which are so obtrusive in the French *savans*, and their English imitators.[67]

The following paragraphs outline physiologic concepts vis a vis digestion in the stomach, the role of a gastric solvent, i.e., hydrochloric acid, the transport of absorbed "aliments," the role of bile and the liver in digestion, and gastrointestinal gas and mucus, all as envisioned at the dawn of the nineteenth century. The descriptive anatomy of the abdominal viscera was more advanced than the physiologic knowledge, and crude microscopes had been invented which had already, by 1800, allowed some delineation of the microscopic structure of the gastric layers. Cuvier had, by 1807, published in France[68] comparative anatomic descriptions of the gross digestive tract anatomy of various invertebrate classes of animals, including crustacean, insects, etc. Observations on the anatomy of the whale stomach were presented in 1808 by Mr. Home,[69] who concluded that

> the first stomach of the whale is not only a reservoir, but the food undergoes a considerable change in it (and that) ... the bones of (ingested fish) must be reduced to a jelly in the first stomach (and that) it is obvious, that as the stomachs of carnivorous animals are the most simple, animal substances, on which they feed, require a shorter process to convert them into chyle than vegetables....

Figure 40 illustrates an 1810 etching, depicting the gross anatomy of the abdominal viscera. A complete collection of engravings of the thoracic and abdominal viscera was published in 1814 by Alexander Monro, Professor of Anatomy and Surgery at the University of Edinburgh.[70] Observations in France by the famous Xavier Bichat on the physiology of the mucous membranes were reviewed in 1821,[71] as well as detailed analyses of the normal vascular appearances of the human stomach.[12] Dr. T.C. Speer, of Bath, presented in 1818 a good description[13] of the vagus nerves, "par vagum," which innervate most of the digestive tract. However, these important parasympathetic nerves, which we know today to constitute the tenth cranial nerves, were described by Dr. Broughton as the "eight pair of nerves over the organs of respiration and digestion."[72] These important gut nerves had originally been identified by ancient physicians as early as Rufus and Galen.

Actual digestion of foodstuffs remained mysterious to physiologists in the early nineteenth century. Many theories had been advanced, from that of Hippocrates who thought food was softened by a sort of putrefaction, or Galen's notion that food was ripened and softened like fruit beneath the summer sun by the great heat of the stomach. Pringle had promoted the concept of digestion by fermentation, Haller by maceration, Borelli and Keil by the mechanical action of the stomach grinding and bruising the food, and all of these early, pre-1800 writers were ignorant of a solvent fluid in the stomach. The discovery of this "solvent fluid" was one of the great advances in physiology which occurred during the first quarter of the nineteenth century; it was first hinted at by Cheselden before this time, and later proven by experiments of Reaumer, Stevens, Spallangani, and others.[73]

Digestion was considered by Glover, in 1800, to depend in man upon the "united causes of solution and fermentation."[74] According to John James,

> the three portions of the alimentary canal, are each accompanied by assistant organs, and each portion performs a distinct part in the process of

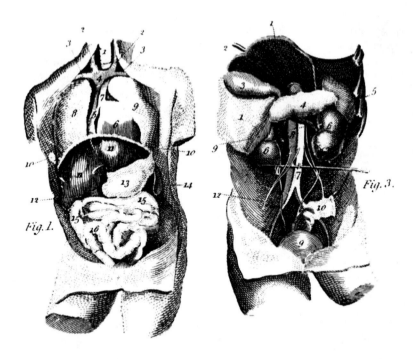

Fig. 40. Gross Anatomy of the Abdominal Viscera. (Etching published by Rev. J. Joyce in 1810, London.)

digestion. The lacteals of each portion, or compartment, are supposed to possess an electric power, by which they select their appropriate fluids — the digestion of one portion does not produce aliment fit for another portion, and when the partially digested food is hurried along the canal with too much rapidity, it becomes, from error of place, offensive and foreign.[75]

Dr. James, in his *Essay on Indigestion*, further elaborated upon the normal physiology of digestion, in which he proposed three factors as operating: chemical powers, mechanical, and most importantly, vital processes.

By an inexplicable vital operation, the digestive system possesses the power of appropriating to the necessary uses of the animal economy a certain and proper proportion of the alimentary matter presented for its election. It is vain for us to attempt to explain this animal and vital process, by an application to it of mechanical principles, or the relations of chemical affinity. The gastric solvent, when made the subject of experiment and chemical analysis, is found to be inadequate to its supposed important agency, and the parietes of the alimentary canal do not possess sufficient muscularity, or strength, to admit of a comminution of food, as has been supposed, entirely or principally mechanical. Yet it cannot be denied that the chemical affinities of the gastric juice, and the mechanical power of the stomach, do in a slight degree aid the digestive process.[75]

James, placing a limitation on the experimental process, further alleged:

> Vitality is a principle beyond the scope of our investigation. No analogy will justify us in degrading the phenomena of vitality, by a comparison with the results of chemical experiments, where the ingenuity of man feebly attempts to imitate the works of his Creator.

James did note that in dogs that had devoured hard cylindric bones of animals,

> if the stomach be laid open a short time after they have swallowed them, the bony fragments will be found divested of phosphate of lime, and may be cut with a knife like macerated horn. It is true this result appears like the effect of a chemical decomposition, and we can apparently imitate this process by subjecting the bones of animals to the action of dilute muriatic (hydrochloric) acid.[75]

Various French writers also discussed digestion,[76,77] and it is interesting to mention some of the specific misconceptions held by several other authors. Cooper and Philip contended:

> Another fact of great importance is, that the stomach is incapable of digesting food when it is diluted with water, beer, wine or any other fluid, which must all be removed before digestion can proceed. This was proved by the fact, that in opening the stomachs of animals, the food is always found comparatively dry in proportion to its distance from the entrance into the stomach, and when it is passing out of the stomach in a digested state, it is uniformly in the form of a thickish paste, whatever may have been the quantity of drink previously taken.[73]

Another error was that of Yeats,[47] who believed that food was "propelled by the action of the intestine and *in part by that of the diaphragm during respiration.*" Others, including Darwin, Fodera, et al.[78] thought there was a direct communication between the stomach and the urinary bladder, without finding it in the thoracic duct, the latter which was conceived by many to be the main route of transfer of absorbed foodstuffs. However, Home had undertaken a number of physiologic experiments with dogs and had proved by 1811 that materials could be absorbed from the stomach directly into the blood stream, and that only a portion of dietary materials passed into the thoracic duct.[79]

The physiologic nature of human gastric juice, as stated above, was debated for many years prior to 1800. Modern reviews on the history of this interesting subject have been published elsewhere.[80,81] By 1800, Harrison had reported a case history[82] of a human showing that swallowed iron nails were partially dissolved by the time of fecal appearance, and had confirmed this experimentally with a dog fed cast iron nails in liver. The "extraordinary powers of the human stomach" were also shown in the case of an American seaman, William Cumming, who swallowed knives.[83] After his autopsy following an extended period in this risky occupation, "fourteen knife blades and number of back-springs were found in his stomach; all of them much corroded, and some nearly dissolved." This "gastric solvent" had been proposed and experimentally verified by earlier workers, as shown in Table 14. John Richardson Young, a pioneer American physiologist was the first to report and prove, in 1803, the presence of acid in the human stomach, as delineated in his M.D. thesis of the University of Pennsylvania.[84]

William Prout was the first to prove that the acid in the human stomach, shown by Young, was actually muriatic acid (hydrochloric acid), and he reported this in 1823 at a paper read at the Royal Society in London.[85] Prout had studied anatomy at Edinburgh under Alexander Monro, referred to earlier in this chapter. However, his training in chemistry under the famed Thomas Charles Hope was the background that had enabled him to chemically identify HC_1 in gastric juice. It was debated between Dr. Adams, Mr. Hunter, and others, around 1810, whether "the solution of coats of the stomach never takes place, except where the person had been suddenly deprived of life,"[86] and this problem of autolysis, during life, is still a central theme which has vexed the understanding of the early etiology of peptic ulcer disease. The composition of gastric juice, at 1813, was also thought by some to contain coagulated albumen,[87] and today we know that gastric juice does contain soluble albumen. Dr. Graves, in 1825, showed that gastric juice contained mucus, "a free acid not volatile," phosphate of lime, and one or more salts containing muriatic acid.[88] In 1808, it had been claimed that gastric juice contained *acetous acid*.[89] Mr. Hunter had proposed that gastric juice was "probably the same in all animals, whether carnivorous, granivorous, or herbivorous ... and that nothing but its life preserves the stomach from digestion."[90]

In addition to in vitro studies of the gastric juice and its digestive powers, and studies on experimental animals which could be sacrificed, at the beginning of the nineteenth century a couple of rare opportunities arose in which human subjects accidentally acquired open fistula into the stomach. Unlike the usual cases of this nature, where the victim would soon die, these cases survived for long periods, allowing physician-experimentalists to study gastric function. The most famous of these was the now-classic case of Dr. William Beaumont (1785-1853), a United States Army physician who studied the fistulous patient, Alexis St. Martin. Although Beaumont's medical training took place in the first quarter of the nineteenth century, his in-depth account of gastric physiology, as undertaken on experiments, began in 1825.[91] His classic findings will not be reviewed in the present chapter, because they fall beyond the selected time period of this book. To Beaumont has usually gone the mass of credit and worldwide historical honor of undertaking the first observations on gastric digestion, based upon carefully designed experiments, in the conscious, "healthy" human.[81,92] However, scientific progress is usually made by a long series of small steps by independent workers. Without seriously detracting from the very notable accomplishments of Beaumont, it must be acknowledged that digestion due to gastric HC_1 (muriatic acid) had already been described, and a prior human with permanent gastric fistula had already been studied and reported by Jacob Anton Helm in 1801 and 1803.[93] Helm had the good fortune to obtain a woman patient named Theresia Petz, of Breiten-waida, a village near Vienna, in 1798. She had a fistula of the stomach, and he studied her until her death in 1802. Though Helm's scientific contributions with his patient were less than Beaumont's work (carried out when chemistry was more advanced), Helm ascertained the temperature of the human stomach, measured the quantity of saliva produced during a normal meal, and studied digestibility of various foodstuffs. Helm's findings were reviewed by Benjamin Waterhouse in 1808.[94] It is of interest to illustrate also, an 1818 view on another case of fistulous stomach:

> Professor Lombard related the case of a man who was wounded by a small-sword, which penetrated the stomach. A fistulous opening kept up a communication between the internal surface of this organ and the external surface of the body, by which channel the patient could, at pleasure, discharge the contents of the stomach, when he found he had eaten too much. What would some of our London Epicures give for such a convenient safety-valve![95]

Other writers besides Helm attempted to elucidate, experimentally, digestibility of various foods, by gastric juice. Scudamore described, in dog experiments, relative digestibility of several kinds of meat, cheese, bone, etc.[96] The times for various foodstuffs to remain within the stomach were described in France in 1818 by Dr. Lallemand.[97] Specific gravity, "solid matter," and "saline matter," were analyzed in chyle in dogs after animal versus vegetable feeding, by Dr. Marcet.[98] The gross description of gastric and intestinal mucus was described in 1823 by Andral,[99] as well as the microscopy of the human gastric surface (greater than 15X magnification, by means of "Mr. Bauer's magnifiers").[100]

The normal functions of the liver, pancreas, gall bladder, and bile duct were reviewed by Benjamin Rush in 1805 in Philadelphia.[101] At this period of time various opinions had been entertained by physiologists in respect to the "office of the liver." Some writers supposed that the secretion of bile was

> merely excrementitious; others that the bile is intended to stimulate the intestine, and to produce a ready evacuation of the faeces; and another opinion has been, that the bile is poured out into the duodenum, that it may be blended with the chyme, and, by producing chemical changes to it, convert it into chyle.[102]

Professor B.C. Brodie supported the latter view, which though nonspecific enough to be noninformative, is partially correct. Chevreul discovered and reported the presence of "cholesterine" in human bile in 1824.[103] Dr. Eaglesfield Smith thought that the fluid secreted by the stomachs of animals did not possess any digestive power whatever but that "the bile is well known to be a powerful animal soap and in its caustic-quality consists its digestive power."[104] Hepatic functions beyond biliary secretion were recognized by 1801, and Powell knew that to a limited degree, the liver could assist in regulating the circulation of blood.[42]

The physiology of gastrointestinal absorption was limited, in the early nineteenth century, by the poor understanding of the chemical breakdown products that were absorbed, by the lack of assays to study absorption, and by the use of test agents that were toxic to animals in absorption studies. Toxic agents used included ferrous sulphate, lead acetate, mercury, and the astringent, nutgall.[105,106] In Pennsylvania, John Hahn had studied the use of enemata to introduce drugs into the body and to hydrate patients. Magendie, the prominent French physiologist, studied absorption in animals,[107] and the controversy raged as to whether intestinal absorption occurred through mesenteric veins or exclusively through lymphatics,[108] although both of these routes were becoming acknowledged.[65] At this early era in medicine, the classic report by Claude Bernard on the role of pancreatic juice in lipid absorption was still to appear, later in 1856.[109]

Chapter IX

Influences of Weather, Lunar, and Other Factors on Disease

It is with more than a little irony that a modern medical scientist should comment upon the holistic, almost superstitious views in which medical scientists of the early 1800's associated disease with environmental factors. From the time of Aristotle, and perhaps before, weather and other factors were thought greatly to influence disease, and this position began to be subjected to scrutiny by the neo-scientific inquiries of the early 1800's. The influence of these factors, described in early nineteenth century literature, has been grossly discarded until recently during the modern era of twentieth century medical science. In the modern era more specific causes such as bacterial, viral, chemical, specific genetic, degenerative or other factors have been found for many human diseases, and are being sought for all. The irony mentioned above lies in the fact that modern epidemiologic investigations, based upon coordinated international comparative studies, sophisticated statistical methods, etc., have begun to indicate in recent years that environmental factors do indeed play a modulating effect on disease. Further, modern laboratory investigations are showing that many diseases seem to be multifactorial, and that whether or not a specific agent causes a disease may be dependent upon a variety of interacting factors, some of which may be general environmental conditions. Thus, in current times we are witnessing international medical conferences in *bioclimatology*, experiencing popularity of *environmental biology*, and increased interest in the field of *geographic pathology*. Although lunar effects on disease (seriously considered in the early 1800's) are not currently taken seriously, and the role of weather on disease incidence is still unproven and poorly investigated, careful epidemiologic studies have shown valid seasonal and regional differences in disease incidence and mortality, and the influence of weather may yet become documented. Titles of a type of scientific papers, such as one presented in the 1970's at the World Congress of Gastroenterology in Copenhagen[1] — "The relation between barometric pressure and the incidence of perforated duodenal ulcer" — are becoming more common. Thus, in the interpretation of the early nineteenth century medical literature we should hold a sympathetic perspective of their theories on the "remote causes of diseases and fevers." A fundamental difference exists, however in the perspectives and logical approach to the interaction of disease processes and environmental factors as used by twentieth versus early nineteenth century medical scientists. In the earlier period inductive reasoning was employed; from specific case histories physicians frequently tried to determine the specific weather or other factors that were *generally* causative of this disease. In the present period deductive reasoning is usually employed; from analyses of general patterns of disease responses on large populations, specific environmental factors are sought which might help explain why an individual patient ultimately develops a disease.

Influence of Weather on Disease

The opinion generally prevailed during the early nineteenth century that temperature, atmospheric pressure, and humidity greatly influenced both animal and vegetable systems.[2] Such influences were of course readily noted with respect to plant life, and, though admitted by the nineteenth century scientists themselves to be less understood, animal functions appeared to be altered as well. Seasonal epidemics had been recorded for many years prior to the 1800's, and cholera had been classified as a summer and autumnal disease, certain coughs a winter disease, measles — an autumnal malady, etc. Further, pleurisy, rheumatism, gout, "angionse affections," "herpetic and leprous disorders" were considered as spring diseases, and summer was thought to bring colics, vertigo, delirium, diarrhea, and gastric and bilious fevers. June, July, and August presented, in Paris, the greatest number of maniacs.[3] Some writers of this early period, such as Dr. Wood of Newcastle, categorically stated that certain diseases derived their origin directly from the state of the weather. Dr. Wood[4] separated those diseases he believed originated from a state of the weather, e.g. typhus fever, from others such as scarlet fever, which appeared to be transmitted by contagion. Epidemics of the latter disease had been noted to be spread by afflicted individuals and epidemics were observed in London, Edinburgh and Newcastle in the autumn of 1806 and in most other cities during the early 1800's. Persons with disease were frequently removed to houses of contagious fever for isolation. Although not understood at the time, we now know that typhus, which was highly fatal in its epidemic form, was in fact transmitted from person to person by the body louse (*Pediculus humanus corporis*) which carried the causative microorganism, *Rickettsia prowazekii*. As a matter of fact the incidence of typhus probably was influenced by seasonal changes, since overcrowding, which would have been positively correlated with congestion in buildings in cold weather, contributed to the spread of this disease.

The respiratory diseases were amongst those thought to be caused or altered by the weather. Dr. Thomas Buxton, Physician to the London Hospital and Surrey Dispensary in 1810 stated[5]:

> It is now so generally understood that many of our English complaints arise from the climate, that we cannot wonder if the means of obviating its inconvenience has very much engrossed the attention of the medical public.... Such is the state of the continent that an English invalid can find safety in no part. The island of Madeira seems now the only spot on which the panting phthisic can feel the balmy influence of an atomsphere suitable to the tender state of the lungs.

Dr. Buxton[5] noted that he had never experienced a spring without losing a number of elderly patients from "active inflammation attacking the lungs" after the "winter-cough" had been present for some time. He mentioned that "the patient catches cold, most frequently at the close of winter, or the commencement of spring." The symptoms he described were characteristic of pneumonia and pulmonary tuberculosis. In order to stabilize the atmospheric temperature in the patient's room to prevent such problems, Dr. Buxton presented detailed plans for the construction of an iron stove which would keep the patient's chamber at 60–65°F. It was reported, further, that catarrh presented "as an epidemic, the effect of the change of weather"[4] and produced a severe fever, termed at that time "influenza," or produced pulmonary symptoms, termed "phthisis." The search for the cause of the common cold, still a popular pastime today, existed even in the early 19th century. Dr. Wood[4] stated in 1808,

> how common it is for every one to try to find out *how they get a cold*, not considering that it is often a general effect of the weather. At the same time, I do not mean to say, that such an affection may not easily be produced, independent of any general effect of the weather; and, vice versa, that by proper management it may often be prevented.

Another disease, characterized by Drs. Fothergild and Wood as an *asthenia* with accompanying "fatigue, weakness of the stomach, palpitation of the aorta descendens, dyspnea," etc., was interestingly theorized as resulting from altered conditions of atmospheric electricity. It was allegedly proven but actually speculated that this malady occurred when the "earth was very much deprived of its electricity, and that it was the deficiency of this powerful agent in the animal economy which produced the symptoms and state of Asthenia...." Dr. Wood asserted that in times of hot, dry and fine weather the earth gave electricity to the atmosphere by means of vapour which partially returned to the earth by means of rain or lightning. A not unreasonable assumption derived by gross observations at that time! It was noted[4] that an epidemic of asthenia, which occurred in May during the fine weather,

> was somewhat relieved by a thunder storm, but not totally, until we had a rain for many hours, on the 31st of the month. The symptoms being less felt in a morning, when the electricity had been partially supplied during the night, and increasing towards evening, when the electricity was again exhausted by means of the day, as well as perhaps by that portion in our bodies being exhausted by exercise.

A further example by Dr. Wood was supplied to support his theory[4]:

> A medical friend of mine informed me, that he was seized with asthma in the evening when returning home from a journey in his carriage, and that he had not had an attack of it for many years; he was relieved by inhaling the vapour of concentrated vinegar. When therefore we consider what share oxygen has in producing the galvanic power, one modification of electricity, *and go round the circle*, we would be led to suppose that electricity itself is oxygen modified, and thus account for the relief my medical friend experienced from the vapour of vinegar, which too may be a likely method of supplying the system with a power similar to electricity.

Because of the significant effects of weather on disease assumed by medical practioners of the early nineteenth century, great attention was given to regional differences in disease incidence. One writer from Dublin, a Dr. Speer, commented in 1822 of the marked and rapid variations of temperature in Dublin, amounting occasionally to 20–30 degrees Fahrenheit per 24 hours, "so that we often have seasons of the day."[6] However, the summer and winter extremes of temperature being cited as less in Dublin than in London or Paris, and the greater regularity of the winds in Dublin were considered as advantageous to good health. The rainfall and particularly the relatively high humidity as measured by the hydrometer were carefully recorded daily for Dublin since the year 1772. Attempts to measure wind velocity by a primitive anemometer were also made by meteorologists of the early nineteenth century and these records were carefully studied by Dr. Speer with reference to diseases he observed in his clinical practice. His conclusion can be summarized by his statement[6]:

> Such, therefore, being the general peculiarities of our climate, it remains for us to inquire how far they are concerned, or what influence they may have in the production of disease. Under the head of temperature we must look to its vicissitudes alone; we must look to the seasons at which these vicissitudes most prevail, — but we find them occurring at all seasons and periods, and must accordingly be prepared for them. It is the order of phlegmasiae that seems here chiefly affected; inflammation is the general character. Sudden changes of temperature will produce more or less sudden determinations to particular organs, and thus the balance of circulation will be more or less distributed and deranged.

This brief statement of Dr. Speer, in a sense, epitomizes the whole of the early nineteenth century perspective of medicine, i.e., the central role of inflammation in disease processes, a concept originating with the school of Broussais, the integration of effects on organ systems with the circulation playing an important role, and the "objective" searching for mechanistic models, either by experimentation or by observations of experiments of nature. Commenting upon the specific role of humidity, Dr. Speer cautiously stated that "how far humidity, unaccompanied with severe cold or heat, contributes to the production of disease or health, is as yet a point not clearly settled." He nonetheless supported the view of others, including Dr. Rutty's paper published in 1772, that moist seasons were the healthiest and most free of epidemics. Stretching his credibility somewhat he suggested that "a single proof of this seems to have been furnished in the year 1816, which was remarkably healthy and remarkably wet."[6] As mentioned above, the spring season was considered to be most unhealthy for respiratory disease, and in Dublin Dr. Speer noted that this was the principal high risk time for inflammation of the lungs, pleura, bronchia and throat, and that acute inflammation of the muscles and joints followed sudden applications of the cold and damp in the spring. He felt that the heat of the summers in Dublin were too mild to produce much gastric, hepatic or intestinal derangements — "they (heats) may revive lurking disease, but they are not strong enough to create it."[6] Furthermore, Dr. Edward Percival, a noted physician of this period, stated in his paper on the Epidemic Fever of Dublin for 1813, 1814, and 1815 that from the beginning of spring to midsummer was the period of most numerous admissions to the fever hospitals.[6]

Inasmuch as the climate of the British Isles was not considered conducive to recovery of certain diseases because of the nature of the weather, it was the practice to send those few who could afford it, to other European regions for recovery. In 1820 a treatise, *Medical Notes on Climate, Diseases, Hospitals, and Medical Schools, in France, Italy, and Switzerland; comprising an Inquiry into the Effects of a Residence in the South of Europe, in Cases of Pulmonary Consumption, and illustrating the present State of Medicine in those Countries*, was published by Dr. James Clark in London.[3] Dr. Clark examined the comparative topography, climate, and habits of the native people in respect to the prevalence (i.e., a crude, nonstatistical determination of prevalence) of disease, and the influence of climate upon recovery of visiting, invalid Britons. His experience reported in this book led him to form a very low estimate of the beneficial influence of the climate of the South of France and Italy on pulmonary consumption (tuberculosis). Dr. Clark stated that

> it appears to me, then, that the change of our English climate for a residence in the milder ones of the south of Europe, is much more beneficial as a preventive of the disease, then, I fear, it will ever be found as a means of cure of it when formed.[3]

It is interesting to note that although genetic concepts were ill-founded and Darwinian evolutionary concepts were not yet developed (Darwin's expedition on the Beagle began five years later), familial factors affecting disease disposition were suspected in 1820 and Dr. Clark, speculating on the influence of climate, stated:

> In the young and growing members of delicate, scrofulous and consumptive families, however, continued for some winters during that age when the body is attaining its full growth, and when cartarrhal affections are attended with the greatest danger, it (climate) may have great influence in checking the tendency to *hereditary* disease. Even when tubercles already exist in the

> lungs in a state of irritation, a residence for some years in a mild
> temperature, together with the adoption of a proper regimen, may be the
> means of allaying the irritation, and consequently of preventing the sup-
> puration of these tubercles. By a little future attention in guarding against
> the known exciting causes of inflammation, these may long, and perhaps
> for life, remain in a state of quiescence.[3]

Dr. Clark visited and studied Marseilles, Hieres, Nice, Villa Franca, Pisa, and
Rome. He considered Marseilles a poor winter residence, with a cold variable
climate extremely productive of pulmonary disease. His description of
Marseilles, one of the early accounts of geographic pathology, continued:

> Another evil of this place, considered as a residence for invalids, is said to
> be the local configuration of its vicinity, which is extremely confined and
> hemmed in by the neighbouring mountains, and by the thick high
> enclosures of the fields and gardens.

He further commented upon the weather,

> It seems irrefragably proved by the experience of our time, that the climate
> of the shores of the Mediterranean is hurtful to such invalids. I have seen
> a great number of these cases terminate fatally at Marseilles, and, at that
> time, I considered the very dry and keen winds of that place, as the principal
> source of evil; but I afterwards found that the warmer, softer, and more
> humid atmosphere of Nice, was in no respect more favourable to such
> complaints.[3]

Dr. Clark also provided some statistics on the prevalence of "phthisis
pulmonalis," based upon admissions to the naval hospitals of the Mediterranean from the fleet in 1810, 1811, and 1812. From the fleet of 30,000 men, 450
cases of phthisis pulmonalis, and 140 of pneumonia were admitted, showing
a proportion of 1 in 65 with phthisis pulmonalis and 1 in 50 when the diseases
were combined. In concluding his book Dr. Clark protested loudly against the
practice of sending abroad patients in a late stage of consumption.

Reports from Scotland[7] also presented meterologic statistics with the
purpose of correlating such data with disease incidence in 1803. It was concluded from one such report that stomach and bowel complaints in Edinburgh
were high in January, along with a stint of especially cold, damp and snowing
weather, a finding that did not agree with other reports on the association of
gastrointestinal disorders with hot weather of the summer.

In addition to the transfer of invalid patients to southern European
climates, which involved only small numbers of people, the medical practitioners of Western Europe and particularly of England, Holland, France and
Spain were concerned about climatic effects on disease because of their navies
and merchants which travelled around the world, and the need for land-based
military operations in foreign locations. The Spaniards travelling to Porto-
bello or Carthagena, the Dutch to the East Indies, Surinam, Curaçao, etc., the

French to St. Domingo, Martinique and Guiana, and the British travelling to Jamaica, tropical Africa, etc. all contended with the problem of tropical diseases in the early nineteenth century. Dr. James Lind published books and essays on this problem,[8] as well as Dr. Pearson, surgeon for the East India Company,[9] and numerous other naval medical officers. It was frequently noted that a "malignant fever of the remitting or intermitting kind" was an epidemic disease of the tropics. This disease, no doubt malaria in most cases, was thought to be "the genuine produce of heat and moisture" and was considered the "autumnal fever of all hot countries."[8] According to Lind the fatalities of the English in Jamaica were most numerous, the number sacrificed to the climate was hardly credible and "that this island formerly buried to the amount of the whole number of its white inhabitants once in five years," and that

> it is a well known and certain truth, that of such Europeans as have fallen victims to the intemperature of foreign climates, nineteen in twenty have been cut off by fevers and fluxes: these being the prevailing and fatal diseases in unhealthy countries through all parts of the world.[8]

Scurvy, which had been well characterized symptomatically by 1805 and was known at this time to be remedied by lime juice, was not a deficiency disease limited to the tropics, but was said by ship surgeons to differ from the usual scurvy when found in the tropics.[9] As a preventive of "the remote causes" of such scurvy on shipboard, "dry air by means of stoves" was recommended in addition to an abundance of water, bread instead of rice, yams or potatoes (also a source of vitamin C) served to the ship's company with their salt provisions, and fresh provisions of vegetables and fruits (the primary source of vitamin C) where attainable. It was further believed by Dr. Pearson[10] that the "ventilation, which hot climates permit and demand, is a powerful cause why people in them are less liable to the contagious forms of febrile disease." Typhus, considered to be a contagious disease, was classified as either typhus icteroides or typhus navium, the latter form seen in crowded ships and running a different course. It was supposedly improved by "effectual ventilation by windsails and opening the ports of the ship," by personal cleanliness and dryness, by fumigation of ships with nitrous fumes, etc.[10] Although physicians in the early 1800's did not recognize the tropical mosquito (female anopheles) as the carrier of malaria, Dr. A. Pearson did indeed correlate the presence of tropical marshes with the genesis of remittent fever in 1804 although for the wrong mechanism. He stated: "I am doubtful if the genuine remittent fever appears without a previous exposure to the exhalation of marshes, or that from rank vegetation." A latent period of up to a fortnight was frequently noted prior to the onset of malarial symptoms after the ship left its port near a tropical marsh. The chronicity of this disease, with its intermittent attacks between periods of imperfect convalescence, was noted. The pathophysiology of this fever, described in 1804, is of interest:

> The debilitating effect of marsh miasmata is generally recognized, (the sedative effects of hydro-carbonate gas, proved to form a considerable part of them, is well known) and it is probable that the nervous energy and muscular irritability, are much and suddenly impaired by their impression upon the sensorium; the powers of circulating the mass of blood are for a time diminished; from that, and irregular actions of the vessels of different viscera, a relative degree of plethora and inflammation takes place, while, from the excretories being similarly affected, the power which the economy posseses to rid itself of an excess of heat is abated.[10]

Other writers, including Dr. Alder[11] have also commented upon the deleterious effect of bad air derived from tropical marshes. It was stated that the air of Jamaica was so bad that even "metals cannot be kept from rust in it; and that this bad air may affect any place at anytime." It was noted that in the West Indies there was a wind every night from the marshy center of the islands toward the sea, and that "marshes, or other sources of putrefaction, situated towards the middle of Jamaica, may affect a camp or hospital situated near the sea during the night." Contagion was considered to be generally downwind. Pure air was considered the best preventive for fevers and in many cases the best remedy,[12] providing that congestion of the lungs had not gone on to inflammation. Dr. Alder, in his treatise, *Proofs of the Theory for the Remote Causes of Diseases and Fevers*,[12] further delineated his theory on the effects of bad air in the causation of disease. He presented a chronological list beginning from the year 433 B.C., of the great plagues of Western Europe, and the "non-coincidental" occurrence of meteors, earthquakes and volcanic eruptions that were responsible for creating bad air which affected such diseases. He indicated that from the year 1000 A.D. there were seven or eight general plagues,

> with the usual attendants, earthquakes, volcanic eruptions, unwholesome seasons, etc. In (the year) 1000 we have the first account of the eruption of Mount Heckla (Iceland). It emitted two meteors like globes of fire. These were followed by severe earthquakes in England, by a very cold winter, and in summer by fluxes, epidemics and mortal fevers. In 1004 an eruption of Heckla and a violent earthquake. In 1005, earthquakes in Italy for three months. Then a famine and plague over the whole earth for three years ...

His list continues like the foregoing, through the year 1798. His citations also include epidemics fatal to cattle and other farm animals, such as the disease of cattle, Angina Maliga, noted in 1682 in Italy, Switzerland, and Germany. The spread of this Angina Maligna epidemic travelled at a rate of half a mile per hour, which was attributed to its causative agent being spread by air. The slowness of its progress allegedly showed either that the cause of it was "heavy and confined near the ground when the current of air could affect it but little; or that the air was calm, or both."[12] Further, the immense meteor noted in March, 1719 was considered the forerunner of the prevalent fevers in Europe that year. There indeed seemed to be no exception to the simultaneous occurrence of large epidemics and natural disasters, in the view of Dr. Alder of the early nineteenth century, who was supporting the hypothesis previously advanced in Webster's *History of Epidemics*.[12]

The role of the atmosphere on disease was thought not, however, to be limited to inhalation of contagious factors, or exposure to undesirable temperatures or humidities. Its effect of pressure on the body surface was also to be considered. In 1802 a report appeared in the *Medical Repository* describing a newly invented machine for "relieving disorders of the human constitution by diminishing the pressure of the atmosphere upon it."[13] This device, invented in England, was capable of removing the weight of the atmosphere upon the leg or arm and was allegedly effective in relieving or curing gout, rheumatism or other painful diseases. The beneficial operation of this machine was said to be aided by admitting watery steam or other vapors into the partially evacuated receiver, a copper vessel, within which the limb rested. The device was sealed at each orifice by a purse-string, ox-bladder seal, and was evacuated by an air-pump. The editor describing this apparatus attested, "It would be a curious process to try what would be the effect of a diminished atmosphere upon the human constitution in certain diseases; and it would be agreeable to have correct accounts of some well-devised experiments to that effect"[13] — another example of the belief in the empirical approach, developing in the early 1800's.

Lunar Influence on Diseases

The belief that the moon and its various phases had profound influence on both normal physiologic functions and disease processes was not unique to the early nineteenth century. Notable medical writers from Hippocrates, Galen, Van Helmont, to Darwin, Mead, Balfour, Lind, Wilson, Leake, and others of the late eighteenth and early nineteenth century had attested with great conviction the role of lunar influence on health. Indeed, treatises on this subject appeared in this period, such as Mead's *De Imperio Solis et Luna*,[14] Folwell's *Observations on the Influence of the Moon on Climate and the Animal Economy; with a proper Method of treating Diseases under the Power of that Luminary,*[14] Balfour's *Treatise on Sol-Lunar Influence in Fevers,*[15] and Bell's *On Periodicity and Lunar Influence in Diseases.*[16] While most writers publishing on this subject believed in such phenomena and had no dearth of examples to support their convictions as illustrated below, a few skeptics existed. An editor of the *Medical Repository*, while admitting to general influences of specific lunar periods on diseases, questioned such relationship[14]:

> We have not the least doubt of the commencement and termination of the many diseases enumerated by the author (Fowell) within the (lunar) periods; but there does not appear to us to be that logical deduction of these from the phases of the moon, at the full and change, that is necessary to con-

vince his readers of their catenation and dependence as cause and effect. There may be, and often is, coincidence without causation.

It is also of general interest in this context that great skepticism prevailed against astrology during this period. "Judicial astrology" was deemed "a vain and delusive art" in this empirical period. It was said that "this calculation of nativities, and the delineation of their horoscopes, have become unfashionable, and have been generally deemed foolish, since astronomy, from a collection of desultory facts, has been improved to a science."[14]

It was reasoned in 1801 that since the moon's attraction had been found to cause the tides of the ocean, that it likewise would induce periodical movements or tides in the atmosphere, which had been shown above to influence, allegedly, health and disease. Thus, a power which could influence the whole mass of water and air must surely have been able to operate upon the bodies of men and animals in some degree! Because of such beliefs the term "lunacy" for insanity and "moon-struck" for madness became common. The manner in which the moon was thought to exert its influence on living organisms was not limited to its "attractive power on the fluids" of vegetable and animal bodies, "a question of ... difficult solution," but also was dependent upon the influence of its light. To some investigators the moon's radiance was a matter of great importance.[16] Others were more cynical, as indicated by a reviewer of Folwell's treatise on lunar influences; as shown here[14]:

> But the moon's magnitude in all her positions remains unaltered, and it is her light alone which suffers enlargement and diminution. To this object the attention of the author, and of other philosophical observers, may be directed with a prospect of usefulness and advantage, through triflers and sciolists may discourage them by remarking, that the grave subject of their researches is nothing but a *matter of moonshine.*

It was accepted, nonetheless, as a fact of nature by many sailors, fishermen, butchers and housekeepers in the early 1800's that exposure of animal matter to the moon's beams accelerated putrefaction. Sound fish were thought to be rendered soft by exposure to a few hours of moonlight and fishermen were careful to cover fish they had caught at night. A mechanism to explain this phenomenom was forwarded; moonlight was thought to produce a greater formation of dew and precipitation of moisture on exposed articles.[16] It was also commonly believed by mariners in the early 1800's that to sleep with the face exposed to the moon's beams would result in swelling of the face and eyes and partial blindness. Indeed, many earlier writers (e.g. Pliny) had described diseases of the eyes of cattle (moon blindness) attributable to the certain phases of the moon.

According to Folwell's account, published in 1798,[14] healthy people were affected by lunar powers.

> Persons in health appear to drink more at the full and change (of lunar period); a plethora is induced in the system; the appetite of

> thirst is much increased, and, perhaps, one-third of usual quantity of liquor is required to make a man drunk at this time.

Further,

> the determination to the alimentary canal is diminished, while that of the insensible perspiration of the body is much increased; the quantity of fluids in the vascular system is more considerable, (and) impressions made on the senses exicite quicker sensations and reflections."

The assumed influence of lunar powers on disease processes were numerous. It was contended that attacks and "fatal terminations of febrile disease and of dysentery," delayed bowel activities, and aggravations of various nervous conditions took place most frequently during lunar periods, i.e. 50 hours before and after each new and full moon.[10,17] One example of a fatal case history, showing the role of eclipses and reported by Folwell in 1798, ran as follows: "In Hartford, State of Connecticut, Dr. T. was found dead in the street. He was going from his neighbor's to his own house, January 31, 1794, and on the same day, hour and minute, the sun was in an eclipse, with a new moon."[14] It should not be concluded from this example that early eighteenth century writers were generally prone to draw conclusions from singular observations. In most cases a collection of clinical experiences, however grossly observed, were presented to advance an hypothesis. One observer, Dr. John Bell, wrote with particular distinction, clarity and wisdom in his general treatise on biological periodicity, which primarily treated aspects of lunar influence.[16] Dr. Bell's article, published in an 1825 issue of the *Philadelphia Journal of the Medical and Physical Sciences*, is of great historic interest to modern investigators in the field of biological and circadian rhythms, a field which has blossomed in the 1960's and 70's. Dr. Bell wisely commented, with respect to the influence of the sun and moon on nervous affections:

> It is natural to believe that these causes exert a feeble action, and that it may be altered by accidental circumstances. But, because in some cases it is not evidenced, we are not therefore to deny its existence. We are so far from understanding all the agents of nature and their diverse modes of action, that it would evince little philosophy to deny phenomena, solely because they are inexplicable in the existing state of our knowledge, though we ought to examine them with an attention the more scrupulous, as the difficulty of admitting them seems greater; and it is here that the calculation of probabilities is indispensable to determine to what extent we must multiply observations or experiments, in order to obtain in favour of the agents, which they point out, a probability superior to the reasons which we may otherwise have for admitting them.[16]

Might not this same philosophical logic apply to the current analysis of highly scrutinized "questionable phenomena" of extrasensory perception, unidentified flying objects, abominable snowmen of the Himalayas or creatures of Loch Ness?

Other maladies believed to be exacerbated by lunar changes included chorea or St. Vitus's dance, apoplexies and vertigos. Wounds of the head were considered most dangerous at the full moon, and attacks of asthma were most frequent especially in the last quarter or after full moon. Fluor albus, which lasted for years in some women, reportedly often had regular returns at every new moon, the discharge lasting some days. Further, nephritic paroxysms frequently observed lunar periods and many cases were on record of "fits of the gravel and suppression of wine every full moon." Tumors were reportedly found to vary in size according to the lunar periods, and hemorrhagic diseases, either primary or vicarious, were thought to follow lunar influence. One striking case reported by Dr. Bell concerned a Captain Richard Boyle of the 3rd regiment of the English guards, and afforded "one of the most decisive examples of lunar influence in medicinal history." The patient was attacked in London, 1785, with pulmonary hemorrhage, and in the following year he was advised to go to the south of France. His clinical history exhibited regular attacks of hemophysis

> on the very day, or within a day of the new and full moon, from February to August, in the different parts of France and England where he was at these respective epochs. The last three haemorrhages came on at the instant the moon appeared above the horizon. Even when the haemorrhage was stopped, the expectoration was as constantly streaked with blood as the moon made her revolutions.[16]

Fevers and mental diseases were amongst those most generally thought to be influenced by the moon. It was said that

> on the mind it (the moon) produces the most powerful effects; as an equanimity of temper, a disposition to cheerfulness and an aversion to anger in people of irascible dispositions. Perhaps there may be discovered in the atmosphere a mixture of airs, at the periods, favourable to the intellectual faculties.[14]

Epilepsy was assumed by a large percentage of practitioners in the British Isles and the new United States to be regulated by lunar powers, and the mentally ill (lunatics) were thought to elicit their manic, affective states in phase with lunar periods. The French physicians remained relatively skeptical of the moon's agency in disease, however, tending to believe that other influences of the night, such as the recumbent position of sleep or sleep itself might be of greater influence. Thus, they felt that the horizontal position invited greater congestion of blood in the brain with accompanying increased susceptibility to epileptic seizures or apoplexies.

It would appear that the politics of science crept into the medical journals of the early nineteenth century even as it does in modern times with respect to selectivity of articles published. An article on lunar influences entitled, "Memoir on a periodical difficulty of breathing, tending to prove the influence of the moon on the human body," was published by D.A. Tranzieri in 1802 in the *Medical and Physical Journal of London*.[17] This contribution, of little value, occupied a full eleven pages of the journal for a single case history, which was excessive even by the permissive journalistic standards of the day. This was permitted no doubt because Dr. Tranzieri was Physician to the Royal Family and President of the Royal Academy of Madrid, and his patient, Donna Maria-Francisca de Parte-Arrozo y Avendanno, was widow of an official of His Majesty's Council and Secretary for the Affairs of India!

Environmental Factors in Disease in the New United States of America

In the new United States of America the views on environmental influences on disease closely corresponded to those in the British Isles; indeed, many of the older physicians in this country had received medical training in the old country. During the early 1800's several medical schools had been established along the eastern seaboard of the United States of America, a country of about 10 million people, at that time, and several medical journals were published with regularity. Dr. S. Colhoun, publishing in the *Philadelphia Journal of the Medical and Physical Sciences* in 1821,[18] summarized the general health characteristics of the American people with particular attention to the regional climatic differences, as well as to the constitutional variances of Americans observed regionally. After characterizing in detail the weather of the United States, Dr. Colhoun stated:

> The winds from the north and west, rendered severe in winter, by passing over extensive regions of snow, descend over the inhabited territories, exalt the tone of the system, and produce inflammatory disorders. During their prevalence, catarrhs, quinsies, pneumonies, consumptions, colic, asthma, gout, rheumatisms, continued and intermittent fevers in an acute form occur.

Furthermore he stated:

> Diseases of a low type in this country, as in Europe, have been supposed to result from prevalence of moisture; united with cold it renders inflammatory diseases more frequent and protracted, and less susceptible of depletion; with heat, the air becomes pestilential, ordinary intermittents degenerate into typhus, and continued fevers become malignant, followed by dropsy and the various forms of nervous debility.

Other writers, such as Bradstreet[19] in Massachusetts, also felt

> that the malignant diseases of our (U.S.A.) hot seasons are arrested by frost, and that even other complaints, common to the summer and autumn, disappear with the approach of winter, probably ... (was) a matter of general consent ...

The assumed deleterious effect of bad air arising from plant degeneration in lowlands was also accepted by the early American workers. Colhoun,[18] describing the Alleghanies as the principal range of mountains which divided the United States into eastern and western sections and the waters of the United States falling into lakes on the north and into the Gulf of Mexico on the south, attested that the waters produced disease "by the putrefaction of vegetable remains on the shores of rivers and arms of the sea, or by the formation of vapor on the surface of stagnant pools and marshes." He felt that in the northern aspect of the United States,

> at a distance from the ocean and great bodies of water, where the air is cold and dry, where from the weakness of the sun and the unfruitfulness of the soil, incessant labour is necessary, the tone of the system becomes exalted, and the diseases are phlogistic in their type; accordingly ... convalescence is more rapid, dropsies, nervous diseases, obstructions of the liver and spleen, disorders of the alimentary canal and bilious fevers are more rare.

It was further contended[18] that

> in latitudes and situations where the vicissitudes of the atmosphere are great, insanity is supposed to occur more frequently; a circumstance perhaps more properly referred to moral causes which have been particularly observed in the highly civilized communities, which occupy those latitudes where the changes of the air are sudden ... Heat alone is a cause of disease; opthalmia, epistaxis, fever, insanity, apoplexy, and gutta serena, are sometimes the effect of an intense sun ...

Dr. Colhoun did not hesitate to examine the broad perspective of the patient's environment! He evaluated, as modern medical students are still being taught with increasing emphasis, the total socioeconomic background of the patient with respect to their disease. His generalizations would, however, be debated today: "in the north, the people contending with the difficulties arising from a dense population, with minds highly tempered by devotion, are subject to mania, from reverses of fortune, and the effects of religion." No one seemed to be spared, however, for he found "the same causes are rendered more powerful in the southern and middle States by a more ardent temperament, and more luxurious habits." There, religion, "vibrating between the extremes of enthusiasm and licentiousness" enhanced the diseases of the nervous system. Religion was not, nonetheless, entirely bad for the health. He mentioned that "religion and law, by encouraging virtue and industry, by repressing indolence and vice, have a direct effect upon the diseases of every community." Recognizing the harmful influences of regional crowding and of filth, Dr. Colhoun observed that

> cities, towns and villages, according to their extent and the habits of the people, become frequent resorts of disease from defect of ventilation, from uncleanliness and poverty, circumstances immediately referable to moral

causes. Prisons, alms-houses, hospitals, barracks, manufactories and ships, where great numbers of people are assembled, are also the seats of many maladies.

The contention by Dr. Colhoun[18] that *heat alone* could cause disease was not shared by all writers in the early 1800's in the United States. An editor of the *Medical Repository*,[20] writing about the "Atmospheric Constitution and Diseases of New York" in 1818, analyzed the meterological data as correlated with respect to disease incidence, and concluded that "with all the intense heat we have experienced, the season has not been miasmatic, nor have we observed any of the numerous effects from marsh effluvia on the human constitution." This writer further asserted that

> a medical topographist, therefore, can illustrate that important question in the history of epidemics, that *heat alone* of climates or seasons is not deleterious; that the wet condition of the ground is a certain *remote*, and a quantity of perishable or corruptible matters is the *proximate* cause of miasmatic disease.

An important book published in 1815 by Dr. Job Wilam of New England on the subject of spotted fever[21] contained considerable insight into the nineteenth century interpretation of atmospheric thermal and other environmental effects on disease. This writer noted that even the health of Indians was influenced by weather conditions; the American Indians "have suffered even more severely (from temperature changes); as might be expected, since they have not the comfortable lodging, etc. which a people in a state of civilization have." One of the noteworthy contributions of Dr. Wilson was his construction of scientific tables of quantitative (meterological) data for the deduction of his conclusions — a practice just beginning to appear in the early 1800's. Most importantly, his conclusions thus achieved, indicated that "epidemic disease of the most fatal character may arise without either the aid of contagion, or of marsh miasmatic influence on the human body." This is an early example of at least partial progress (with respect to miasmatic influence) in medical science arising from the exploitation of quantitative, analytical study of retrospective data. Wilson's views[21] on the mechanisms by which temperature changes could induce disease are of interest from the standpoint of early nineteenth century pathophysiology:

> Great, sudden, or rapid changes of temperature are considered as the predisposing and exciting causes of the popular distempers in New-England. Catarrh, influenza, and spotted fevers are derived from one and the same source, and are but grades or modifications of the same disease. It is admitted that a single vibration of temperature is insufficient to produce spotted fever, however great and sudden it may be. To accomplish this there must be a series of changes to break down the inherent energy of the capillary vessels, and to destroy to a certain degree this active power. And where this torpor was produced among the people of one of these devoted regions, the characters of it were legible in their countenances, which, as their hands and feet, were more or less of a purplish hue.

As far as can be ascertained from the origin, symptoms and progress of spotted fever, and from dissection after death, the proximate cause would seem to consist in a torpor of the minute vessels of the skin and of the bronchiae; but while the capillary tubes are thus held in a state of atony, there is an overcharge of blood in the lungs, heart, pulmonary vessels, and internal organs. If both the capillaries and large arteries and veins are debilitated in nearly an equal degree, there will probably be no fever; because the equilibrium of excitement and circulation is supported throughout. But when, by reason of atony in the extreme vessels, the balance of distribution is destroyed, there may be too great a mass of blood about the thoracic and internal parts, and an inability to diffuse it regularly through the body. Hence may arise the struggle in the constitution to re-adjust the vital and propelling forces, to equalize the circulating fluids, and to restore once more the impaired functions to their proper condition. A fever is the consequence.

Lunar influences on disease were also seriously considered by the early American medical practitioners, as described by Dr. John Bell.[16] Because of the debates on the nature of lunar and solar effects, Dr. Bell called upon his colleagues,[16] readers of the *Philadelphia Journal of the Medical and Physical Sciences*:

I would solicit the members of the profession, in the various parts of the United States, to keep a register of the sick under their care, the duration of the disease, and of the termination in death. By this means, in a few years such a mass of testimony might be accumulated, as to settle forever the question of sol-lunar influence, and the extent of the periodicity of diseases in general.

Chapter X

Cold Affusions, Cold Water Bathing, and Topical Use of Blisters

General Theory of Animal Heat and Cold Therapy

The role of bathing in maintaining health and in therapy for the sick has long been acclaimed since the beginnings of medical history, both for the salubrious effects of cold temperatures on health and because of the mineral content of spring waters. Hippocrates and Celsus recommended cold bathing, which was used in the treatment of Emperor Augustus.[1,2] Galen described cold water immersion as fit only for the young of lions and bears, but that warm bathing was conducive to the growth and strength of infants.[3] By the early nineteenth century, treatises had been published on the art and powers of mineral waters, modes of bathing, and beneficial effects of cold affusions for a multitude of diseases. In 1820, it was stated:

> Good and evil are almost as intimately blended in the moral and physical world around us, as nerve and blood vessel in the wonderful microcosm within us. If the earth pours forth miasmata that scatter sickness and death among all within their range, she also distils from her secret recesses salubrious springs, to revive the drooping invalid, expurgate the pampered epicure, and dispel those physical sources of melancholy that sap the foundation of human enjoyment, or absolutely abridge the range of life.[4]

Specific directions for bathing, including recommendations not to enter the cold bath when the body temperature was below the standard of health, not to remain too long in water, not to bathe on a full stomach, to bathe in water at 65°F, etc., were published in the early nineteenth century in England and the United States.[5] Many published accounts during the early nineteenth century attested to the presumed importance of external, environmental temperature on disease incidence, ranging from accounts on adverse effects of solar heat[6] and bowel and liver disorders caused by heat to coughs and chest disorders in colder weather.[7] This particular, important notion of weather effects on disease is dealt with in some detail in another chapter in the present monograph. However, an understanding of the endogenous origin of animal heat and its relation to human disease, as perceived by the medical profession in 1800–1825, is helpful in understanding why these physicians resorted to cold affusions, and temperature-regulated bathing for therapeutic purposes.

In the time of Galen, it had been disputed whether animal heat depended on the motion of the heart and arteries, or whether the motion of the heart and arteries was innate but that body heat was not a fundamental property. Hippocrates, the founding father of western medicine, thought animal heat a mystery, and bestowed upon it many attributes of the Deity.[8] Nonetheless, by the beginning of the nineteenth century it was recognized that body heat was generated internally, and although it could be modulated within narrow limits by environmental temperatures, was kept rather constant for maintaining life itself. All physiologists of this era believed that there was a vital connection "betwixt the degree of heat generated, and the state of circulation," and at death the "lifeless mass sinks to the temperature of the bodies around it."[8] Philosophical discussions of animal heat were provided by many early nineteenth century writers, including Dr. Thomas Welsh of the Massachusetts Medical Society, Dr. Dugud Leslie, Mr. Adair Crawford, and others.[8] Leslie believed that blood contained phlogiston, which was activated and set into motion by the action of blood vessels (which were perceived to contract and circulate the blood), and that the evolution of phlogiston was the mechanism by which nature produced heat, whether by friction, tissue inflammation, physical ignition, or normally in vivo. Leslie considered that venous blood was warmer than arterial blood, a concept denied by Dr. Crawford, who believed the converse. Crawford postulated that in respiration the blood continually discharged phlogiston and absorbed heat, and that in the course of circulation, blood imbibed phlogiston and emitted heat. Crawford maintained that during respiration, oxygen combines with carbon, "producing a species of slow combustion, in which a quantity of caloric is extricated," but this chemical view of the process of animal heat was refuted by Dr. N. Chapman in 1823.[9] Welsh hypothesized that during circulation blood gave out heat that it had "received from the air in the lungs; a small portion of this heat is absorbed by those particles which impart the phlogiston to the blood; the rest becomes redundant, or is converted into moving or sensible heat." Dr. John Bell considered the above concept of heat originating from the inspired air philosophically incorrect, and that heat arose from action of the blood vessels. Excessive body heat, such as in fever or from an inflamed part, eventually would evaporate from the body surface as "one of the means employed by nature for moderating the heat, and restraining the violence of disease," and Welsh therefore considered applying cold affusions as facilitating this process.[8]

As discussed above, there was some controversy about the origin and nature of animal heat. William Henry in 1803 discussed the hypothesized materiality of heat, since it had long been a question among philosophers, whether the sensation of heat, and the class of phenomena arising from the same cause, be produced by a peculiar kind of matter, or by motion of the particles of bodies in general ... Since, therefore, caloric is characterized by all the properties, except gravity, that enter into the definition of matter, we may venture to consider it as a distinct and peculiar body ... [and] that heat can subsist independently of other matter, and consequently of motion; in other words, *that heat is a distinct and peculiar body*.[10]

In addition to motion, oxygen gas was conceived to be intimately linked with the origin of heat or caloric. Mr. Tupper, writing on animal heat in 1802, stated that "the blood is formed from animal or vegetable matter, or from both, and, like each of them, abounds in hydrogen and carbon; both these bodies have a strong affinity for the basis of oxygen gas, and when they combine with it, caloric is always extricated." Tupper further elaborated,

> When warm blooded animals are placed in a cold medium, their venous blood assumes a much darker hue than when they are placed in a warmer; for, as the animal heat greatly depends upon the evolution of the heat from the blood, in consequence of its combination with hydro-carbonaceous matter, more especially in the capillaries; so therefore, when animals are placed in a cold medium, they deteriorate more air in a given time than when they are placed in a warmer; and hence it appears, that the quantity of heat which is separated from the air, and absorbed by the blood in the act of respiration....[11]

It was further proposed by Dr. Henry Earle in 1816[12] that the nervous system exerted a significant influence in regulating animal heat. Dr. Earle experimentally showed that a limb deprived of its nervous influence, such as in human patients with limb pain treated surgically by nerve resection, became chronically of lower than normal temperature. Also supporting Earle's belief that circulation of blood was not the sole determinant of body heat, was his observation on vascular ligation, viz:

> When a ligature is placed on the principal artery supplying a limb with blood, the circulation in the smaller anastomosing vessels, and in the capillary system is much increased. The limb is furnished with a smaller quanitity of blood, but what does circulate must necessarily pass through vessels of a smaller calibre, consequently, they are preternaturally distended with blood; and if a limb be examined under these circumstances, it will be found that the communicating vessels are enlarged. They subsequently undergo a further change, and after some time again contract to their former size. The effect produced by these changes on the temperature of the limb, is an increase of heat beyond the natural standard of the healthy limb, at that part immediately below where the artery is tied, which increase of heat gradually extends itself over the whole limb. This could not happen if the temperature depended solely on the circulation....[12]

Some physiologists in the early nineteenth century, such as Gordon, thought that heat was evolved during the coagulation of blood, but others, such as Dr. Hunter and Dr. J. Davy disagreed. On experiments with the blood of sharks or of sheep, Dr. Davy concluded "that during the coagulation of blood, there is no sensible evolution of heat."[13,14]

Interrelationships between the triad of the physiology of body heat, the external or environmental sources of heat, and of disease were described in 1804 by Dr. Pearson of London, who was a surgeon in the service of the East India Company.[15] In an attempt to correlate differences in disease incidence, climate, and body stature with heat, Pearson contrasted the European with the Oriental, viz:

> Among the inhabitants of the more temperate and colder regions of the earth, the natural consitution is that of muscular irritability and promptitude to action; the nervous mobility is not so great, the influence of that power being more equable, steady, and moderate. The solids are denser; of this there is a remarkable proof drawn from the fact, that between an European and an Hindoo or Chinese of apparently equal bulk, the difference of weight is very great, the former being much heavier. The blood contains a greater proportion of crassamentum, and there is also a greater quantity of the circulating mass. The cuticular discharge [sweat] and the biliary secretion [bile] are in smaller quantity; the power of absorption is greater, especially its action in the renewal of the solid parts of the body. The use of animal food and of fermented liquors is more indulged in, and with greater impunity. Such is the natural and the general constitution in cold climates; but adventitious modes of life alter that in very many individuals. Peculiar habits and employments, luxury and sensual gratifications, often induce the temperament of increased mobility and diminished tonic power in them and their progeny, which is in a great measure the same with that which is impressed by hot climates ... [In the cold climate] diseases of inflammation and of excitement will be produced, and are found to occur. A continued exposure to the effects of heat at length induces a different state of the frame ... [and] the ultimate effect is relaxation of the [blood vessel wall muscular] fibre, and an irregular or weakened performance of the functions of the different organs. [The state of health being brought on by residence in hot climates included:] ... a degree of fever becomes habitual, there is a sinking in of the abdomen, wasting of muscular substance, chronical inflammation and scirrhus of the glandular viscera, and painful sensation in parts where no sensation ought to be felt.[15]

Dr. Pearson, after propounding the above philosophy, provided an extensive list of dietary and therapeutic regions for individuals arriving to hot climates, and included cold bathing in his recommendations.[15]

Specific Medical Uses of Cold Affusions and Cold Water Bathing

The range of medical maladies which were therapeutically treated by either cold affusions or cold water bathing in the early nineteenth century was quite extensive. These organic and constitutional diseases, birth defects, or toxic drug reactions so treated included almost the gamut of observed medical problems, some of which would seemingly benefit from cold treatment with a logical basis, such as fever or burn reactions, and others which did not. The latter maladies included such problems as hydrocephalus, abdominal hernia, and insanity. The multitude of published case histories, expounding the salubrious benefits of cold therapy, demonstrate the fact that such treatment truly elicited dramatic patient responses which were recorded. As is the case with many nineteenth century therapies, we can conclude that some of the recoveries would have happened spontaneously anyway, and that positive, beneficial placebo responses would also be observed as they are today observed.

In the case of acute reactions of cold water therapy, the nonspecific shock effect may in many cases have overridden any response specifically related to body temperature reduction. The overt and dramatic human response, of well or sick patients, to dousing the head with cold water was not a unique observation in any case.

Rheumatism and gout were treated with alleged effectiveness by cold water immersion of the affected limb. In Smith's popular book entitled, *Curiosities of Common Water* and in Rigby's treatise on *Animal Heat*, the local application of cold water for relief of gout was recommended.[16] Sometimes this treatment was managed by the attending physician, who would order the local soaking of the gouty limb in cold water or who would wrap the affected limb with wetted cloth, soaked in cold water.[17] In other cases, the salubrious effect of cold water on gout pain was recorded following patient directed demands, such as the interesting case reported in 1804 of a superintendent of a fishery in Newfoundland.[18]

In this case the afflicted victim demanded to go to sea in a fishing vessel, against the wishes of his friends,

> by crying out that his pain and the heat of the affected part were so great, he was confident nothing could abate them but cold; and if that did not relieve him, he would prefer to die at sea as suffer so much torment in bed. The consequence was, that the poor sufferer was carried to the vessel, in which he put to sea, and was obliged, as is usual, to remain for several hours nearly up to his knees in salt water.* In this situation, to the great astonishment of everyone present, the pain and inflammation abated, and the man ceased to complain; on his return home he insisted on his wet clothes remaining upon him, and in case of the symptoms returning, to have buckets of sea water in readiness. By this treatment he always procured relief; and his habits of living induced many severe accessions, almost every year, for which he would be carried into the sea and there remain until the accustomed alleviation of his symptoms took place; besides this, he had the inflamed parts wrapped in cloths immersed in the same fluid, which never failed of procuring the desired relief.

The present writer, who has resided in Newfoundland, can readily attest to the coldness of these North Atlantic waters, a sea which occasionally freezes in winter and is chilled even in the summer by the cold Labrador current.

Topical application of cold water was used for generalized acute rheumatism, and was considered a safe and beneficial mode of therapy. Wetted clothes reportedly produced the relief of joint pain, and bathing in cold spring water was associated with reduction in rheumatic pain.[17,19] One physician who became afflicted with severe acute rheumatism in every joint of his body and who acquired "the odious appellation of 'the lame doctor,' " rid himself of his "vexatious companion, rheumatism" by immersions into cold spring water, relief he did not find by attempts at dwelling in a hot climate or by use of drugs. His discourse on this beneficial therapy was summarized in 1803:

> I determined to try the effect of immersions into cold spring water. I continued indefatigably the use of the immersions for nearly four months. I constantly bathed once, frequently twice, and sometimes three times a day. At each immersion, I usually swam about in the water for a few minutes. For the first month the bathing seemed to have no other effect upon me than a remission of rheumatism while I was in the water. In the course of the second month, I was more encouraged to proceed in my cold plan. At last I relinquished the bathing, because it was unnecessary to seek further for what I had already found, *a perfect recovery*. It may be proper to observe, that during the bathing I adopted the use of fleecy hosiery stockings, which I believe materially assisted in the completion of the cure.[19]

Application of cold sea water, sometimes in combination with zinc sulfate (a drug which is still used today as an agent to promote healing, and has been reported by the present author to inhibit experimental gastric ulcers, in part by mechanisms related to inhibition of the release of intracellular enzymes[20,21]) was reported in 1815 to facilitate the healing of leg ulcers.[22]

The use of cold water, obtained by melting snow, was recommended for the acute treatment of scalds,[23] a therapy which apparently was rivaled by use of the heated oil of turpentine[24] in 1806 in the United Kingdom. Dr. Dzondi analyzed the mechanisms by which he believed cold temperature aided the burn lesion[25]:

> The cold, if it operates in continuation, has a double effect on all organic bodies; it deprives them of a part of this caloric (heat), lessening thereby their distension, increases contraction, and of course brings the parts into closer contact. In this manner it removes the too great warmth of the burnt part, lessens the unnatural distension and pain, increases the connection of the parts, contracts the vessels and the cellulosa, prevents the accumulation of the fluids, and thus operates in opposition to the heat.

In addition, Dr. Dzondi suggested that cold partially or totally suppressed the "vital activity" of the organism and reduced the sensibility and activity of the nervous system, thus alleviating pain, mechanisms with which we would find little to argue with today.

Strangulated inguinal hernia was treated successfully in 1807 by affusion of cold water to the affected region, allowing immediate relaxation and reduction of the hernia.[26]

Opium poisoning, a problem manifest by profound stupor, was effectively treated by cold affusion to the head and chest.[27] Large bucketfuls of cold spring water, "forcibly thrown on the head and chest" roused the stuporous patient, allowing subsequent treatment with an emetic. This therapy was reported by several physicians in 1823.[27]

In Germany, Professor Heim, a celebrated physician of Berlin, treated children with "evident congestion of the brain," accompanied by lethargy or coma, by cold water application to the head. He recommended[28]:

> ... the hair being first removed, that a piece of cotton or many threads of worsted should be twisted, and applied as a band round the head, in the course a saw would be directed in an anatomical examination: this precaution ... prevents the water from running off too fast, and coming on other parts not intended to be cooled. Then the child being placed across the lap of an attendant, with its head projected, and the face downwards, ice-cold water is to be poured, by means of a funnel, from a height of six inches or a foot, round, and on the head. This should be continued unceasingly for a quarter of an hour at a time; therefore a third attendant should be ready with plenty of the prepared water. The running water may be received in a vessel placed under the child's head. The part should then be wiped dry, and the child put into a moderately warmed bed. In about an hour the affusion should be repeated, and so continued for twenty-four hours; the second day it is repeated in the same way every two hours; the next, at longer intervals; and is thus persevered in till the child recovers or expires.

In the early nineteenth century in England cold water application to the head was employed for the treatment of madness, "apoplexia mentalis" or insanity. Dr. Brown of Bath placed a handkerchief around his patient's head, kept it wet with cold water, and persevered with this treatment for up to 15 days, whereupon the rationality of his patient returned.[29] As mentioned below, warm water immersions were also used in the treament of insanity.

A variety of infectious diseases were treated by cold affusions, in large part because these diseases induced severe fever which was counteracted by cold water. Typhus and scarlatina were treated by sponging the body not only with cold water, but with vinegar as well.[30] In 1807 fifteen cases of typhus, treated by cold water affusion, were reported in Derbyshire, England. One patient, with a burning skin and pulse rate of 110 was "taken out of bed, placed in a tub, and (had poured upon him) two buckets full of cold water...," a treatment followed by cure of the patient.[31] The description of this series of fifteen cases of typhus ended with the optimistic belief in cold affusion, viz:

> All the patients took bark and wine, and opiates and opening medicines, as occasion required; but I am inclined almost to attribute every thing to the reduction of the temperature of the body by cold water; and I most gladly and confidently join in the opinion, that the true remedy for typhus is simple, and at hand; that it dwells in every fountain, travels in every stream, and murmurs in every rill.[31]

Also smallpox was treated by cold water affusion at four-to-six hour intervals,[32] as was colic.[33] Tetanus, which produced severe muscular spasm, was treated by cold water shower baths with alleged success.[34,35,36]

Other convulsive diseases, which in the nineteenth century would have included a multitude of infectious diseases in which high fever ultimately progressed to convulsions, were also treated by cold affusion. Dr. Dewar described[37] the efficacy of cold well water affusion used on British troops stationed in the Mediterranean. A number of soldiers of the Queen's Regiment of Foot arrived at Minorca in July, 1800, by frigate, but soon elicited intermittent fever. Sixteen men, on the average, were taken ill each day. They were removed from bed, stripped, and doused with cold water. Dr. Dewar mentioned, when he had the occasion to apply this procedure to females, "their delicacy was saved by allowing them to retain their shift, which was changed immediately after the operation." This procedure provided an immediate relief "from the head-ache, from the heat of the skin, and all the symptoms of pyrexia." Dr. Dewar returned to England, impressed with the effect of cold affusion:

> Knowing the present spirit of enterprise which prevails in the medical world, I expected on my return to this country in 1802, that the cold affusion must be universally employed, and was rather mortified to find, that though no facts were brought forward to its discredit, many medical men seemed very unwilling to employ it.

In the early nineteenth century, fevers were known to have many origins, and fevers were classified as intermittent, remittent, low autumnal, bilious, or dysenteric fevers, and fevers associated with local affections, and inflammatory or eruptive fevers. Dr. Robert Jackson, while in Savannah, Georgia, became himself a victim of fever probably arising from malaria and he reported on his beneficial use of cold water affusion, and drinking of cold well water for fever therapy.[1] Amongst his views on the treatment for fever, reported in 1808, he considered

> bleeding as the most important, whenever there appear marks of local congestion, inflammation, or that sluggish and torpid action which marks incapacity in the circulating vessels ... Emetics and purgatives are advised for the same purpose. All these are considered under certain circumstances, as preparatory to the great remedy of cold affusion.

Others expounded also that cold affusion would "carry off, by evaporation, the superfluous caloric" or excess heat, and published dissertations on "the cold practice in febrile diseases," including Dr. Vine Utley of Connecticut and Dr. James Currie of Liverpool,[38] and Dr. Charles Shilleto of Surrey, who practiced the sudden immersion of patients into the sea.[39] Many other writers of this period, including De Haen, Gregory, Gerard, Brandreith, Wright, M'Lean, Dimsdale, and others recommended cold affusions for fevers of all types.[40,41]

Observations on Hot Bathing, a Converse Therapy to Cold Affusions

The early nineteenth century rationale for use of cold therapy was based upon its observed, apparent beneficial effects, espoused in the current medical journals and treatises, and was rationalized as a benefit for removing excess heat, or for other actions such as shock effects. Why then, would the opposite treatment, that of hot bathing or local exposure of affected parts to heat, be rationalized for many of the same diseases? A partial answer to this paradox has universal applicability to medicine, historical and modern; ignorance generates speculation and diverse schools of thought. Dr. A. Nicholl, of Edinburgh, assistant surgeon to the 80th Regiment and fellow of the Royal College of Physicians, tested young men to determine at which warm temperature a bath was salutory, and at which temperature it became injurious to sick or healthy subject.[42] He placed his subjects in a bath at 86°F–110°F, or affused them with warm water, and monitored pulse rate changes and body temperature. His physiologic findings were reported in 1818, and he noted that baths "above the standard of the human body are injurious, more particularly in cases of fever. Warm immersions (first 98°F, then 107°F) and warm affusions on the head were characterized as relieving insane persons in London in 1814.[43] The drinking of hot water was used to overcome hysteria.[44] Hot vapor baths were used with salubrious effects in patients with tetanus, by Dr. Marsh of Ireland,[45] and a portable hot vapor bath device was reported in 1814 by Jennings in the United States of America,[46] who used heat conducted by a pipe from this vapor bath as a sovereign remedy for fevers. Nonetheless, his method was not commonly accepted, as most physicians preferred the use of cold. One case history, reported in 1825, attested the most harmful effects of hot water bathing, extended for six hours, for treatment of chronic rheumatism.[47] In this report,

> A charlatan advised the patient to remain immersed, for the space of twelve hours, in a hot bath, the temperature of which he gradually raised very nearly to that of ebullition. She entered this bath at mid-day, and remained in it six hours, when she lost all recollections; an hour afterwards she was found entirely deprived of feeling, with her head supported by a board covering the bath. She was immediately taken out of the water. The face was enormously swollen and blackened; the eye-lids tumefied; the eyes distorted; the skin was of a dark-red colour, burning, and bloated; perfect loss of feeling and recollection; taciturn delirium; grinding of the teeth; foaming at the mouth; convulsions of the limbs; increased on the slightest touch; respiration laborious and rattling; abdomen distended, particularly at the epigastrium; pulse hard, concentrated, frequent, and irregular.

It is no wonder that extreme, hot bathing such as the above case, was ill-advised. However, it remains unclear why predicted beneficial responses to mild heat, such as in cases of arthritis, were not noticed, and why the harmful chilling effects of cold water soaking for extended periods were not more often recorded in nonfebrile cases.

The Therapeutic Uses of Blisters and Related Topical Appliances

The practice of applying irritants topically to the body is one of great antiquity. It was employed in the early nineteenth century both on local affections such as sore joints, and also at some distance from the malady with the belief that internal disease might be brought from deeper disease organs to the surface of the body, and dispelled. Local irritation of the skin by use of blisters, wrappings which contained irritant chemicals, were believed to be able to draw the congestion fluid of diseased organs to the skin. As well, relief of deep pain by substitution of the lesser pain of a superficial irritant, the principle of counter-irritation, was noted after use of blisters. This latter phenomenon is still observed today, and is practiced by the laity with patent medicines, though is usually not recommended by physicians because of the availability of analgesics of superior effectiveness. Blisters have also been used with great popularity in veterinary medicine, particularly in large animal practice for limb and joint wounds.

The term, "blisters," arose because the irritants would actually elicit blisters upon the skin. In the early nineteenth century "plasters" were used, which were bandages containing less irritant chemicals, and a "vesicating plaster" was a blister which contained a potent irritant, such as the powder of cantharides. Blisters were frequently applied for extended periods of days or weeks, and as a result the underlying skin would desquamate. In all probability in the early nineteenth century, occasional benefits were actually observed (i.e. pain relief) after use of blisters, but many of the improvements would have occurred spontaneously anyway by normal healing processes, and we can surmise that often more harm than good was done.

Dr. Aaron Dexter, reporting in the *Medical Communications of the Massachusetts Medical Society* in 1813,[48] recommended the use of a vesicating plaster of cantharides for treatment of diseases of the articulations. He followed the advice of Mr. Samuel Cooper, of the Royal Surgeons in London, who had received a prize in 1806 for his treatise on treatment of large joints. Cooper has advised

> in the strongest terms, large blisters sufficient to cover the diseased part, and the surface to be kept open with the savin ointment steadily applied, till the cure is effected, without any regard to its cause; and that fomentations and poultices are totally unworthy of our attention; for, if they do no harm, an insidious disease is gaining ground, which sometimes proves fatal to the life or limb of the patient, by neglecting severe measures, as soon as they are indicated.[48]

Nitrous acid was at times employed instead of a bandage-type blister to produce an immediate counter-irritation of great severity. This was used by Dr. Killet, an assistant surgeon of the British 3rd Regiment Light Cavalry in Madras in 1821, for treatment of "spasmodic cholera." It was published that the great good effects of this sudden and powerful counter-irritation (two parts acid and one part water, rubbed over the surface of the abdomen) were strikingly illustrated in the case of a European, who received immediate relief in the burning sensation at the stomach on the acid blister being applied; and who, the next morning, being annoyed with spasms of the extremities, requested the same remedy might be applied; it was accordingly done, and so great was the relief obtained to one leg, that he cried for God's sake to apply it to the other, similarly affected.

This use of nitrous acid application for counter-irritation was considered a great convenience, and it was felt

with this remedy in our hospitals, it should no longer in urgent cases be observed in the journals, that the "blister did not succeed," or "the blister was applied, but could not be kept in its place, for no circumstance can prevent the application of the acid, and its action, when applied, cannot possibly fail.

Also, according to Killett, blisters were used

in those cases of severe disorder in the stomach and bowels, consequent on excessive drinking, where the promptitude is of vital importance, and where common blisters are altogether useless and inapplicable; also in cases of acute and sudden pain from other causes, in hepatitis, and so forth; wherever the disease depends on spasm, or nervous irritation, the relief is wonderfully sudden; and when it is connected with inflammation, I think it is fully as certain, and more speedy, than after common blisters.[49]

The dermatologic response to nitrous acid, though harmful as described below, was thought to be less dramatic than that to blisters; viz:

Whoever has felt the tedious progressive pain of a blister, the wearisomeness and irritation produced, and the agony of motion; the sickness and disgust of the dressing, and the after sickly smell, itchiness, etc., will be disposed almost to suffer any pain rather than submit to a repetition; it is obvious, that all these circumstances must have their bad effects on the patient.[49]

The dermatologic aftereffects of cantharides were also severe, as described by Dr. Killett in 1821[49]:

If the acid has been diluted with half its bulk of water, and applied lightly with a feather, the cuticle is stained of a straw or sulphur colour; in three days it begins to pucker, with a little serum underneath; a slight red ring surrounds the parts, and the cuticle comes off on the 4th or 5th day, leaving the surface like a common blistered part, with a few deeper streaks, where the cutis vera has been touched. But if the acid has been used undiluted, or has been longer applied, the cuticle becomes of a deep brown; it does not rise or pucker, as the subjacent vessels necessary for throwing it off, appear to be destroyed; the red ring forming on the 3rd day becomes deeper and broader, and a portion of the true skin, of the thickness of sheep's leather, begins to separate in six or seven days. The parts are rather tedious in healing, but this, taking it in all its bearings, is no great disadvantage.[50]

In part owing to the type of adverse tissue reactions described above, it is not surprising to note that the entire medical community in early nineteenth century Britain, Europe, and the United States did not endorse the use of blisters. Syer of Warwickshire stated that the administration of blisters was something "upon which the medical world is a good deal divided."[51] He had only "very faint hopes of the utility of blisters beyond the third or fourth day of any acute universal disease, characterized by severe topical inflammation." Syer thought "perhaps the only contra-indication to the use of a blister, is that of extreme irritability." The well-known Dr. Kinglake suggested[50] that in cases treated by blisters, "most of the instances would, probably, have recovered without blistering, as they are found to do with it," and

> that vesication over the cavities in inflammatory affections of the subjacent viscera, has at once greatly aggravated the local disease, and the general irritation usually on these occasions pervading the system ... Where unnatural torpor and deficient re-action exist in diseases, the stimulating effect of blistering may usefully excite the languid and drooping state of life; but, on the contrary, where excessive irritability and violent excitement present, the additional stimulus imported by vesication would appear to be contraindicated and necessarily harmful.[50]

Amongst those physicians who felt postively toward the medical use of blisters was one J. Augustine Smith, who was in 1809 professor of anatomy and surgery in the University of the State of New York, as well as member of the Royal College of Surgeons of London. In the treatment of a case of a dislocated and probably broken leg (which he predicted would likely result in loss of the female patient's leg), he applied a blister, two inches wide, encircling the entire leg which was by this time swollen and vesicated.[52] The patient's leg recovered, which Dr. Smith attributed to the beneficial effect of the blister, which "arrested the process of mortification."

Dr. Matthew Baillie of England treated a case of hydrocephalus, which caused the unusual separation of the skull bones in a seven year old boy, with the combination of a large blister applied to the scalp, as well as internal administration of mercury, squills, and digitalis. Eventually, the patient died.[53]

The well known Sir Gilbert Blane reported in 1815 in London the efficacy of the use of very large blisters in treatment of "cynanche laryngea," a disease with chronic inflammation and suppuration of the larynx, but which cannot be identified with certainty at the present date.[54] Sir Gilbert stated:

> From my own practice, and that of others of equal experience with myself, there is great room from analogy to place confidence in blisters of a large size in this disease; for in the inflammation of other vital parts, the bowels

NOMS des MALADIES.	CURATION										
	EXTERNE.					INTERNE.					
						Boisson		Injection			
	Bains	Douches	Fumigations	Lotions	Pédiluves	Martiale	Sulfureuse	Axale	auriculaire	Urétrale	Vaginale
Adiapneustie, SAGAR	46	»	»	20	»	»	9	»	»	»	»
Agrypnie sénile	40	12	»	40	»	»	6	6	»	»	»
Aménorrhée	56	»	35	»	45	15	15	»	»	»	30
Ankilose	35	24	60	25	30	»	12	»	»	»	»
Atrophie	60	20	»	70	24	»	18	»	»	»	»
Boutons (phyma, SWEDIAUR)	45	»	»	120	»	9	9	18	»	»	»
Cachexie	60	»	»	45	»	»	36	6	»	»	»
Cancer	72	»	24	40	»	»	12	»	»	»	»
Dartres	96	»	56	30	»	16	50	20	»	»	»
Engelure	19	8	»	»	»	»	3	»	»	»	»
Entorse	28	25	»	»	»	»	9	»	»	»	»
Epilepsie	51	18	»	60	25	»	15	15	»	»	»
Exarthrose ischio-fémorale	25	20	»	»	»	»	6	»	»	»	»
Galactoplania, SWEDIAUR	96	»	36	»	40	8	10	27	»	»	»
Galè	45	»	»	95	»	»	18	»	»	»	1
Goutte	76	55	»	»	»	9	33	»	»	»	»
Haemoplania, SWEDIAUR	45	»	»	»	36	»	12	16	»	»	»
Hémorrhée	8	»	»	»	6	»	3	»	»	»	»
Hidroplania, SWEDIAUR	96	26	»	»	»	»	45	»	»	»	»
Lèpre scorbutique	72	»	»	96	»	»	48	»	»	»	»
Menoplania, SWEDIAUR	48	»	24	»	36	»	12	»	»	»	»
Ménorrhagie	56	»	»	72	»	»	18	»	»	»	»
Obstruction (1)	3,195	1,217	412	705	800	236	403	950	»	18	65
Ophthalmie	190	»	180	»	»	»	54	»	»	»	»
Paralysie	260	185	»	»	»	»	39	»	»	»	»
Phthisie	36	»	»	»	40	»	9	»	»	»	»
Rachitis	28	16	»	»	»	»	6	»	»	»	»
Rhumatisme	460	128	80	»	»	»	90	»	»	»	»
Scorbut	96	»	»	»	»	18	24	»	»	»	»
Scrofules	160	»	»	»	»	»	36	»	»	»	»
Stérilité	80	»	48	»	»	12	18	»	»	»	45
Surdité	36	»	»	»	»	»	12	»	24	»	»
Tumeur blanche	60	»	»	»	»	»	12	»	»	»	»
Uroplania, SWEDIAUR	16	»	»	»	»	»	5	»	»	»	»
Vomissement idiopathique	35	»	»	»	»	16	6	»	»	»	»
TOTAUX	5,807	1,755	955	1,462	1,082	339	1,091	1,058	24	18	140

Fig. 41. List of numerous maladies treated in 1822 in a French hospital, by internal or external application of mineral water. (Des maladies traitées aux eaux minérales de Bagnoles [Orne], sur des maladies des deux sexes, de tous les âges et de toutes les conditions, pendant l'été hippocratique de 1822.) Published in "Mem. de Méd., de Chir. et de Pharm. milit." 16 (1823) 270.

and lungs for instance, I can say from undoubted experience that I have seen the most striking success from blisters covering the whole thorax or abdomen, in cases similar to those in which small one had failed. The effect of large blisters is indeed so different from that of small ones, that they may be considered as a distinct class of remedies. In the present complaint it does not seem necessary that the blister should be directly over the part affected, which does not afford sufficient space; nay a better effect may rationally be expected by the application being made to the neighbouring parts, for the inflamed organs are so closely subjacent to the external surface, that the stimulus of the blister and the afflux of circulating fluids consequent upon it, might even prove hurtful. It is observed in inflammations of the eyes, that a blister at some distance is more beneficial than one very near....[54]

Ileus, or intestinal colic was treated by a large blister over the abdomen.[55] In general, for symptoms with

active inflammation, general blood-letting is advisable, and safe to a greater extent than is commonly practised, locally also by cupping or leeches; fomentations, blistering over the seat of the pain, and dressing the blister with mercurial ointment; above all, by mercurial purges given in repeated doses....[56]

Chapter XI

Quicksilver and
Other Materia Medica

It is likely that in prehistorical times ancient man attempted to cure his diseases or relieve discomfort by many means, including the ingestion or application of nonfood substances to his body. Although this point cannot be verified, there is no doubt that since the dawn of recorded history, man has continually attempted to treat therapeutically his ills by medicines, whether they be effective, ineffectual, or even iatrogenic. In primitive societies, where traditions have been handed down only by word of mouth, medicines have been widely used, and were often administered along with magical rites. Even in current times, primitive or "folk medicines" remain in use in both underdeveloped and sophisicated societies, and are even increasing in popularity, due more to fads than to a rational or logical basis. In primitive times in the western world practically every imaginable vegetable, animal or mineral product, however noxious, has been used as a medicine. The virtues of materials ranging from dried horse or dog excrement, to turpentine have been extolled, and still today in traditional Chinese medicine, peculiar biologicals ranging from powdered antlers to pulverized insects remain in use. Of course, most of such materials or their extracts contain a complex of chemicals, some of which may possess significant pharmacologic activity, as well as toxic or even carcinogenic or tumor promoting properties.

The nineteenth century view that "sick persons should feed on noxious substances" was inherited from earlier times, and indeed detailed noxious medicinal regimens have been recorded and promoted since early historical times. The Ebers papyrus over 3,500 years ago listed more than 700 medicinal products,[1] and a few of these compounds have remained in use as a result of empirically-proven effects on the human body. Some of these early noted agents include alcohol, tobacco, caffeine-containing beverages, marijuana, opium, and the quinine-containing bark of the cinchona tree, or "Jesuit's Bark," which was an effective anti-malarial agent. The most ancient known Greek physician, Melampus of Argos, allegedly cured one of the Argonauts of sterility by "rust of iron in wine," and the daughter of King Proetus of melancholy with "black hellebore," an opium or veratrine preparation. In the *Iliad*, wounds were treated by surgical and medicinal means, as:

> Patroclus cuts the forked steel away,
> Then in his hand a bitter root he bruis'd,
> The wound he wash'd, the styptic juice infus'd:
> The closing flesh that instant eas'd to glow,
> The wound to torture, and the blood to flow.
>
> (from the *Iliad*)

Drug Combinations, and Specific Insolation of Compounds

Combinations of innumerable natural products were commonly used from ancient times and well into the nineteenth century. One of the first of these was known as *Theriaca Andromachi*, or theriac. Originally concocted by Nero's physician, Andromachus, in the first century A.D., it was based upon the earlier formula devised by Mithridates VI (126–64 B.C.), King of Pontus in Asia Minor. Galen also created a version of the theriac which consisted of 63 ingredients. Throughout the centuries in Europe many cities, including Venice, Genoa, and Constantinople, were noted for their theriacs and the theriac of the French pharmacopoeia consisted of 71 ingredients in 1837, and of 56 ingredients by 1884.[1] Of course, many of the components of the theriac exerted no real effect.

Though theriacs, herbal and crude preparations of many sorts continued to remain popular during the nineteenth century, the dawn of this century witnessed the beginning of the limited *scientific* enlightenment with respect to drug therapy. This was only a spark of enlightenment at this time, manifest by the chemical isolation of several pure pharmacologic agents and the influence of Francois Magendie of France, who became the founder of pharmacology. It remained for later pioneers in medicine in the late nineteenth and twentieth centuries to implement significantly this rational form of drug therapy, i.e., the use of a pure chemical for a defined and correctly understood physiological process.

Morphine (meconic acid) was isolated from opium in 1805 in Germany by chemist Friedrich W.A. Sertürner, (1783–1841), and several alkaloids, including quinine, brucine, caffeine, and strychnine were isolated from plant material by Joseph B. Caventou and J. Pelletier in France early in the nineteenth century. François Magendie included such compounds in his medicinal *Formulaire*, published in 1821. These purified compounds were not only chemically isolated and applied for human use, they were also tested experimentally on animals. Sertürner found that his crystallized morphine induced sleep and indifference to pain in dogs. Experimenting with himself and three of his friends, with a dose of morphine ten times greater than that recommended today, Sertürner observed that it induced profound depression lasting a few days.

K.F.W. Meissner (1792–1853) of Halle, cooperating with Caventou, isolated veratrine alkaloid in 1818 from the seeds of hellebore (*Schoen ocaulon officinali*), a plant known from antiquity to be poisonous. Veratrine is now known to be a mixture of several alkaloids, and was used as a local irritant and hypotensive agent. These two pharmacologic pioneers also isolated colchicine from the autumn crocus, used from Roman times for treatment of gout.

Pelletier and Magendie isolated emetine from ipecac (*Uragoga ipecacuanha*) in 1822, and named it in accordance with its marked emetic activity. It still remains one of our most useful agents to induce vomiting. Magendie also studied the poison used on arrow tips in Borneo, a substance derived from the *Strychnos* plant, and tested it on dogs and even horses. Magendie noted its convulsant activity, and attempted to study its pathways of absorption and distribution and site of action. Thus, he initiated one of the first scientifically based experiments in pharmacodynamics and pharmacokinetics. His students Claude Bernard (1813–1878) and James Blake (1814–1873) later in the nineteenth century published numerous brilliant experimental studies in medicine and physiology, encouraged by their tutelage from Magendie. In France Magendie had outlined some of the basic premises required for the analysis of drug actions; i.e., the principle of quantitative analysis of dose-effect relationship, the role of chemical and temporal factors in drug absorption and assimilation, the principles of localizing the site of drug action and of drug specificity (later followed up by Claude Bernard), and the principle of chemical structure-activity relationship (later developed by James Blake and others).

The Modus Operandi of Medicines

In spite of the significant beginnings of scientific pharmacology promulgated by Magendie, the generally accepted views on medicines and the therapeutic practices followed by most early nineteenth century physicians were based on simple and erroneous concepts. Dr. Chapman, discussing the mechanisms of drug action in his 1827 treatise, *Elements of Therapeutics and Materia Medica*, stated,

> not a little difference of opinion prevails on this very intricate question. The only point in the controversy which seems to be conceded, is that the operation of medicines does not depend on any of the common laws of matter, but on a principle incident to vitality alone,

viz, *Medicamenta non agunt in cadaver*.[2] Quoting the distinguished Cullen's analysis on the odors of medicines, Chapman divided medicines into the following classes:

Aromatic: Generally stimulant and transiently corroborant.

Fragrant: Analeptic, and sometimes antispasmodic.

Ambrosial: Powerfully so (as fragrant medicines), and likewise cordial.

Alliaceous: Actively stimulant, bracing the nerves, and exhilarating the spirits.

Hircine: Sedative and deleterious.

Stinking: Anodyne and poisonous.

Sickly: Narcotic—though in its primary impression it proves so offensive as often to puke or purge.

Chapman proposed for the operation of medicines "that they all act by exciting a local impression, which is extended through the medium of *sympathy*." He considered the other view, held by his contemporaries,

> By many, however, it is still believed, that certain articles, at least, enter the circulation, and produce their effects in this way. The last hypothesis is evidently a relic of the humoral pathology. By the disciples of that sect, it was held, that disease mainly consists in a depravation of the blood "from too great tenuity or viscidity—by an excess of acid or alkaline acrimony, by morbific matter entering from without, or generating within." As a necessary consequence of such notions, medicines were supposed to penetrate into the circulation, and by a sort of chemical action, to correct the vitiated condition of the fluids, and hence the origin of the terms, inspissants, attenuants, antacids, antalkalines, antiseptics, diluents, demulcents, etc.

Professor Chapman had classified, by 1827, drugs into emetics, cathartics, enemata, diaphoretics, diuretics, lithontriptics and antilithics, emmenagogues, and expectorants. Specific examples of emetics and cathartics, as outlined by Chapman, are listed in Table 15.

In his debate against the contemporary theory that drugs acted through circulation, Chapman stated that should

> more proof be required of the operation of medicines being independent of the circulation, it might be found in the well-ascertained fact, that many of them produce their full effects, though the heart and blood vessels be previously removed. Long ago it was shown by Whytt, that if the heart of a frog be taken out, and a solution of opium injected into the abdomen, the animal speedily becomes convulsed. The poison of the viper, according to Girtanner, applied to a frog prepared in the same way, will destroy it as soon as if no mutilation of the animal had taken place.

On the converse side of the argument, Dr. Brodie had contended

> that corrosive sublimate kills by acting chemically on the mucous coat of the stomach. But arsenic, emetic tartar, and the muriate of barytes, by entering the blood. That alcohol, the essential oil of almonds, the juice of aconite, the empyreumatic oil of tobacco, and the woorara, operate through the nerves, without being absorbed into the circulation. But the woorara, applied to a wound, communicates its effects to the brain, by entering the circulation through the divided vessels.[2]

Table 15
Classes of Therapeutics and Materia Medica*
(Professor N. Chapman, 1827)

Particular Emetics
Callicocca Ipecacuanha
Spiraea Trifoliata
Euphorbia Ipecacuanha
Sanguinaria Canadenesis
Nicotiana Tabacum
Lobelia Inflata
Scilla Maritima
Antimonium
Antimonium Tartarizatum, vel Tartis
  Antimonii
Sulphas Cupri: vulgo Cuprum
  Vitriolatum
Sub-sulphas Hydrargyri Flavus:
  vulgo Hydrargyrus Vitriolatus
Zinc Sulphas: vulgo Vitriolum
  Album

Particular Cathartics
Ricini Oleum
Olivae Oleum
Sulphur
Magnesia
Cargo Vetetabilis:
  vel Carbo Ligni
Sales Neutri, or Neutral Salts
Hydrargyri Sub-Murias, vulgo
  Hydrargyrus Muriatus Mitis
Rheum Palmatum
Convolvulus Jalapa
Aloe Perfoliata
Cassia Senna
Cassia Marilandica

Popophyllum Peltatum
Juglans Cinerea, vel Juglans
  Cathartica
Convolvulus Scammonia
Stalagmitis Gambogioides
Helleborus Niger
Cucumis Colocynthis
Cucumis Agrestis
Croton Tiglium

Enemata
Diaphoretica, or Diaphoretics
Diuretica, or Diuretics
Lithotriptica et Antilithica, or Lithontriptics and Antilithics
Emmenagoga, or Emmenagogues
Expectorantia, or Expectorants

Particular examples are listed only for emetics and cathartics. A number of these plant or chemical substances were still in use in the 1950's, but of those, high toxicity has been ascertained and modern substitutes now exist. Some of these agents, such as Croton Tiglium *are now known to be cancer promoting. Lists are extracted from Chapman.* [2]

By the *medication* of the blood, moreover, were it possible, I insist that we must in all instances do harm. The whole mass of circulating fluids is equally charged in this case with the medicinal substance, and, therefore, while an action is going on in a diseased organ, which may be salutary as to it, every sound part of the system becomes exposed to a similar impression, which could not fail to disturb the order of health, and create morbid derangements. If it alleged, as it sometimes has been, that the action of medicines, under such circumstances, is on the surface of the blood vessels, or through the connection which the blood has with the solids, the doctrine becomes deserted, and we are forced to recur to sympathy, as affording the only explanation. [2]

Pharmacopoeias and Pharmacy Journals

The first official European pharmacopoeia was published in 1498 under the title, *Nuovo Receptario*, in Florence. In subsequent centuries, many pharmacopoeias appeared, representing not only a particular country or city, but, as reviewed by Urdang,[3] reflecting the ebb and tide of various political influences. At the conclusion of the eighteenth century several European pharmacopoeias were in use. In Italy, the *Ricettario*, published in 1789 in Florence, was the official Florentine pharmaceutical standard and its content had remained unchanged for at least a century — only its title page had altered due to the fall of the House of Medici in 1737. In 1790 the Venetian republic broke with the older tradition of publishing in Latin, as the rising tide of Italian nationalism overcame the aristocratic republic of the nobles, and the *Codice farmaceutico per lo stato della serenissima repubblica di Venezia* was published as a formulary in Italian. Soon, however (in 1798), the Austrians seized the Venetian republic and created in 1814-15 in the Lombardic-Venetian Kingdom the *Pharmacopoea Austriaca*. This formulary also replaced the 1794 (Latin) and 1795 (German) *Pharmacopoea Austriaco Provincialis*.

In the United Kingdom the *London Pharmacopoeia* was in use from 1618-1851, the *Edinburgh Pharmacopoeia* from 1699-1841, and the *Dublin Pharmacopoeia* from 1807-1850. The first Spanish pharmaceutical standard, *Pharmacopoeia Hispana* appeared in 1794. In France, where the autonomy of the large cities had earlier dictated that each follow its own pharmacopoeia, e.g. the *Pharmacopoeia Lugdunensis* of Lyon and the *Codex Medicamentarius Parisiensis* for Paris, before the French Revolution centralized the government. Conseqently, a more universal pharmacopoeia for the whole of France was instituted, after some delay[3] and was known as the *Codex Medicamentarius sive Pharmacopoea Gallica* in 1818.

The Netherlands of Belgium and Holland followed similar pharmaceutical standards in the early nineteenth century. The Batavian republic (1795-1806) issued a proclamation in 1803 that "there shall be one pharmaceutical code for the entire Batavian republic according to which all pharmaceutical stores shall be administered." Accordingly, in 1805 the Amsterdam pharmacopoeia entitled *Pharmacopea Batava* served this purpose. This was replaced in 1823, after formation of the Kingdom of the Netherlands, by the *Pharmacopoea Belgica*, as well as by the Dutch *Nederlandsche Apotheek* in 1826. Poland also established an official Polish pharmaceutical standard in 1817, as did Finland in 1819, compendia known as the *Pharmacopoeia Regni Poloniae*, and *Pharmacopoea Fennica*, respectively. In Germany the *Pharmacopoea Borussica* (1799) was the first official pharmaceutical formulary in this country. The first edition of a pharmacopoeia for the new United States of America appeared in 1820, though it represented in true democratic fashion a concensus of medical opinions from diverse nationalities, rather than a nationalistic treatise. Further, it should be noted in passing that the North American Indians themselves possessed an extensive materia medica, which varied from tribe to tribe. A list of the herbal medicines used by these Indians has been compiled by Corbett,[4] and includes more than 72 plants, including flowering dogwood, dandelion, corn smut, blackberry, ginseng, juniper, peyote, white oak, and smooth sumac. Aside from the 1820 American pharmacopoeia mentioned above, other related treatises were available in the new world. The physician-botanist Johann Schoepf had published in 1787 a book, *Materia Medica Americana Potissimum Regni Vegetabilis* about the indigenous American medicines. Also, botanist Benjamin Smith Barton published a two-part treatise on American materia medica in 1789 and 1804, the first of its kind in the English language. In 1808, *Pharmacopoeia* was published by the Massachusetts Medical Society.

The earliest regular journal of pharmacy having a scientific character was the *Journal der pharmacie für Aerzte und Apotheka*, edited by J.B. Trommsdorff. An earlier Germany pharmacy periodical had previously been established in 1780 by Johann Goettling, but appeared only annually.[5] In 1797, the first French pharmaceutical journal, *Journal de la société des pharmaciens de Paris* was founded, which was followed in 1809 by the *Annales pharmaceutiques françaises*. The earliest American pharmaceutical journal to be published was the *Journal of the Philadelphia College of Pharmacy*, which appeared in 1825.

Development of Schools of Pharmacy, Pharmacy Laws, and Hospital Pharmacies

At the dawn of the nineteenth century the regulation of training and requirements for qualifications to practice pharmacy were beginning to receive increased attention. Earlier, in the eighteenth century, the druggist simply compounded and stocked cheap medicines for the poorer people in Europe. However, in the U.K., the London Society of Apothecaries stimulated parliament to pass an Apothecaries Act (1815), designating certain powers over professional standards and education. In the United States of America, similar pharmacy laws were passed for the Territory of Orleans (1808), Louisiana (1816), South Carolina (1817), and Georgia (1825). All other states followed this pattern of the south, later in the nineteenth century.

In France, though, apothecary schools had existed long before, the *Collège de Pharmacie* was established in 1777, and legislation of 1803 provided six higher schools of pharmacy to train first class pharmacists (who could practice anywhere in France), and second class pharmacists (restricted to practice only in districts in which they were examined). The *Collège de Pharmacie* by 1796 had created a new organization, the *Société libre de Pharmacie de Paris*, and a *Société de Pharmacie de Paris* by 1803 to encourage scientific communication and interaction.[5] Likewise, in Germany the pharmacist promoted science and occupied an honorable niche in his society in the early nineteenth century. The great German poet, Goethe, stated in 1822 that "in Germany the pharmacist enjoys a highly esteemed position within society.... The German pharmacists cultivate science. They are aware of its importance and endeavor to utilize it in practical pharmacy."[5]

In North America the first school of pharmacy was established in 1821. It was officially called the Philadelphia College of Pharmacy and Science, but was better known as the Philadelphia College of Pharmacy. This was in the same city in Pennsylvania as the first medical school of the United States of America. Here, as elsewhere, medical schools and pharmacy schools developed in parallel. In 1823 the Massachusetts College of Pharmacy was established.

In addition to training formally in pharmacy schools, pharmacists have had a long tradition of practical training in the hospital and military environment. Modern hospital pharmacy has been considered to have been born in Paris at the beginning of the nineteenth century,[5] and from this time on played a key role in the scientific development, research and publication of drugs and their actions. In England, the hospital pharmacist also served as a medical practitioner, but in France he was involved mainly in drug compounding and research in drug chemistry. In France, pharmacy service for the military hospital, the office of "apothecary-major of the battlefields and the armies of the king," had been established in 1766, and by 1824 this post had become designated as *pharmacien inspecteur général*. Well-known French military pharmacists include J.A. Parmentier (1737-1813), who did research in food chemistry, and Ch. Laubert of Napoleon's *Grande armée*.

Medical Sectarian Aspects of Drug Use

As evident throughout the present monograph, the therapeutic excesses of medical practitioners were clearly manifest in the early nineteenth century, and included all therapies ranging from excessive blood-letting to drastic drug and heroic physical treatments. Understandably, these treatments with potent emetics, purgatives, and other agents (Table 15) instilled a fear among the laity which provided a fertile ground for the growth of sectarian drug treatments which were less offensive. One of these groups was the Thomsonian sect which began just at the onset of the nineteenth century under the leadership of Samuel Thomson. As this was an early American development, it is described in Chapter VI on American medicine. From the standpoint of drug therapy, Thomson's system was based upon earlier precepts of botanic and herbal therapy, though it was unique in that he systematized and patented his teachings.

Although Thomsonians claimed to offer milder and safer botanic therapies, they still continued to recommend frequent medicated enemas, extremely hot teas, etc. The materia medica of the Thomsonians was divided into six classes of drugs, based upon their actions.

Another sectarian group in medicine followed the doctrine of homoeopathy propounded by Samuel Hahnemann (1755-1843) in 1810. This unorthodox pharmacologic system originated in Germany but later was accepted rather widely in the developing United States. Homeopathy truly represented an alternative to the drastic medical therapies practiced by the orthodox physicians in the early nineteenth century, as it was founded on the premise of the *simile principle*. This concept purported that a disease could be cured by remedies that evoke symptoms resembling the disease in question. To induce such symptoms minute doses of drugs were required in order to excite the required type of irritation. This concept of "like is cured by like" without doubt was less noxious and harmful to patients than the kinds and amounts of poisonous agents administered by orthodox physicians. Hahnemann required that his patients be treated only with fresh drug preparations (tinctures), rather than dried agents, and importantly, that only a single active drug be administered at a time.

The Reverend John Wesley, A.M., published in London[7] a booklet entitled, *Primitive Physic: or, An Easy and Natural Method of Curing Most Diseases*. The twenty-sixth edition of this volume appeared in 1807, attesting to its popularity. This book promoted a natural and conservative lifestyle, with recommendations such as[7]:

A due degree of exercise is indispensably necessary to health and long life.

Tender persons should eat very light suppers; and that two or three hours before going to bed.

Malt liquors (except clear, small beer, or small ale, of due age) are exceeding hurtful to tender persons.

All pickled, or smoked, or salted food, and all high-seasoned is unwholesome.

Tender people should have those who lie with them, or are much about them, sound, sweet, and healthy.

Wesley prescribed a number of pharmacologic agents or herbal remedies for specific diseases, as illustrated by the following examples:

For the spitting of blood "take a tea-cupful of stewed prunes, or two spoonfuls of juice of nettles ... or, three spoonfuls of sage-juice in a little honey ..., or, half a tea-spoonful of Barbadoes Tar, on a lump of loaf sugar at night. It commonly cures at once."

For vomiting blood, "take as much salt-petre, as will lie upon half a crown...."

For dissolving coagulated blood, "bind on the part ... grated root of Burdock spread on a rag...."

For boils, "apply a little Venice Turpentine."

For hard breasts, "apply turnips roasted until soft, then mashed and mixed with a little oil of roses. Change this twice a day, keeping the breast very warm with flannel."

For "sore breasts and swelled, boil a handful of Camomile and as much Mallows in milk and water. Foment with it between two flannels...."

> For a burn or scald, apply oil; and strew on it powdered ginger, ... or
> twenty-five drops of Goullard's Extract of Lead, to a half pint of rain
> water....
>
> For a cancer in the breast, drinking twice a day a quarter of a pint of the
> juice of Clivers, or Goose-grass, and covering the wounds with the
> bruised leaves, ... or frequently applying red Poppy water, Plantane,
> and Rose-water, mixed with Honey of roses....

The Dispension and Warehousing of Drugs

The hospital pharmacy, as well as the apothecary shop and in rural areas the travelling drug salesman, the physician himself, and the homemade concoctions such as described above by Wesley were typical sources of drugs in the early nineteenth century. To these sources can be added the special medical chests, such as could be purchased by physicians in London, and as designed for particular uses. The contents of one type of dispensary, the family dispensary, are outlined in Table 16, as available at the Chemical and Medical Hall at 170, Piccadilly in London. The family dispensary chests "neatly made of mahogany, and the bottles of the best flint glass, with airtight stoppers," were available in six sizes ranging from 20 pounds 8 shillings to £6 6s., at the year 1800.[8] The fine quality of ingredients contained in such dispensaries is clearly substantiated in Figure 42, as these agents were sanctioned by the nobility. Other types of medicine chests included: the traveller's dispensary (made flat, for the pocket of a carriage), the tropical dispensary (for the East and West Indies, Africa, and South America), the country clergyman's dispensary (made on a very cheap plan, and supplied with black bottles), the sea medicine chest (for the use of the navy surgeons and captains of merchantmen), the veterinary chest (or gentleman's stable dispensary; see Table 17), as well as other types of chests such as a chest of apparatus (for chemical experiments) and a mineralogical chest.

Drugs were also available from drug warehouses, such as the large enterprise developed in 1807 as a manufacturing and distributing center in Philadelphia (Fig. 43).

Use of Selected Drugs (Antacids, Emetics, and Heavy Metals)

A. Antacids

It is beyond the scope of the present chapter to review in detail all pharmacologic agents in popular use in the early nineteenth century. However, some particulars on a few selected pharmaceuticals will serve to characterize the general state of the art in respect to some aspects of medical therapy in this era.

Dr. Richard Reece, Fellow of the Royal College of Surgeons of

Table 16

Family Dispensary (1800)[8]

Five Bottles in the Back Part, contain

1. Magnesia
2. Epsom Salt
3. Castor Oil

4. Tincture of Rhubarb
5. Cajeput Liniment, or
    Opodeldoc

Five Bottles in the Front, for

6. Comp. Tinct. of Bark, or
7. Tinct. Ginger and
    Camomile
8. Com. Tinct. of Senna

9. Com. Spirit of Lavender
10. Mindererus's Spirit
11. Paregoric Elixir

Nine Bottles in the Right Wing, for

12. Spirit of Hartshorn
13. Spirit of Sal Volatile
14. Vitriolic Ether
15. Sweet Spirit of Nitre
16. Antimonial Wine

17. Tincture of Myrrh
18. Dilute Sulphuric Acid
19. Tincture of Assafoetida
20. Volatile Tinct. of Guaiac
    Gum

Nine Bottles of the Left Wing, for

21. Salt of Wormwood
22. Crystall. Lemon Acid
23. Ipecacuan Powder
24. Essential Salt of Bark, or
25. Salt of Steel

26. Rhubarb Powder
27. Jalap Powder
28. Camphorated Powder
29. Com. Cretaceous Powder
30. Extract of Lead

Nine small Bottles in a Drawer, for

31. Liquid Laudanum
32. Essence of Peppermint
33. Essence of Cinnamon
34. Prepared Calomel
35. Emetic Tartar

36. Basilic Powder
37. Antimonial Powder
38. Camph. Acetic Acid
39. Tincture for Tooth-ache

Six Pots in a Drawer, for

40. Blistering Plaster
41. Spermaceti Ointment
42. Brown Cerate
43. Yellow Basilicon

44. Savin Ointment
45. Squill Pill
46. Aperient Pills
47. Lenitive Electuary

Six Drawers in the Front, with Partitions, for

48. Peruvian Bark, or Rhat-
    any Root Powder
49. Jamaica Ginger Powder
50. Senna Leaves
51. Flaky Manna
52. Gum Arabic Powder
53. Purified Nitre Powder

54. Cream of Tartar
55. Flowers of Sulphur
56. Court Plaster
57. Lint and Plaster Skins
58. Diachylon
59. Ditto with Gum
60. Carbonate of Soda

THE

CHEMICAL AND MEDICAL HALL,

170. PICCADILLY,

OPPOSITE BOND-STREET,

Was established by the Author in the year 1800, to supply the public with *genuine* drugs, and the *choicest* chemical preparations, and to compound prescriptions with accuracy, on the most *reasonable terms.* The practice of adulterating drugs, and of substituting cheap articles for expensive ones, in the compounding prescriptions, &c., which prevails to an alarming degree, renders any observation on the advantages of such an institution unnecessary. The sanction it has experienced from the nobility, and the most celebrated chemical and medical characters in the United Kingdom, he considers a proof of its having been conscientiously conducted.

The Author having received from his friends residing in the East and West Indies, America, and in the country, many complaints of their commissions having been taken to the shops of chemists and druggists to be executed, although their agents were desired to apply to the Medical Hall, he begs to state, that no article is sold there without a printed label, expressive of its name, and of its having been obtained at the *Medical Hall*, 170. *Piccadilly.* This regulation he has adopted not only for the satisfaction of his friends, but for the support of the reputation of the Establishment.

Fig. 42. Testimonial and advertisement as to the high quality of drugs available in medical chests, in 1800 in London.

Table 17
Pharmacologic Agents Provided
in the Veterinary Chest, Available at the Chemical
and Medical Hall, London, 1800, as Advertised[8]

It contains one large Drawer, with Partitions, for

Cathartic balls	Cough balls	Aniseed powder
Strong balls	Alternative powders	Liquorice powder
Worm balls	Nitre powder	Foenugreek powder
Alternative balls	Flowers of sulphur	Antimony powder
Diuretic balls	Cordial balls	Liver powder

Nine Bottles in the Top Part, for

Spirit of wine and camphor	Embrocation for sprains
Spirit of turpentine	Goulard's extract
Opodeldoc	Laudanum
Oil of wild thyme	Distilled vinegar

Four Tin Cases, with Partitions, for

Blistering, or Spavin ointment	Healing ointment
Alternative, or Grease ointment	Mercurial ointment
Cooling ointment	Digestive ointment

Six small Bottles, for

Corrosive sublimate	Butter of antimony
Lapis infernalis	Red precipitate

London, outlined in his *Medical Guide* of 1824 the practical application of many pharmacologic agents.[9] In tables he presented on dose levels recommended for numerous drugs, he outlined doses for children (age 2–4 years) as differentiated from adult doses. His comments on the use of antacids were of particular interest. These agents, which even today remain relatively unchanged, are *almost* as effective and useful in the treatment of peptic ulcer disease as our modern and sophisticated agents, such as histamine H-2 receptor antagonists, tricyclic depressants, etc. The comment by Reece on magnesia as an antacid, including a peppermint flavoring additive and its known tendency as a laxative, remains remarkably correct; viz,

> This article (magnesia), by neutralizing acid matter in the stomach, speedily relieves the painful sensation termed *heart-burn*, and with it forms an aperient (laxative) medicine, which operates gently on the bowels. The dose is from a tea-spoonful to a desert-spoonful. It operates most pleasantly when administered with an aromatic, as peppermint-water, or with two grains of ginger-powder or grated nutmeg in spring-water.

However, on the basis of modern medical knowledge, Reece's physiologic explanation of the mechanism of how magnesia operates is completely wrong. He believed that "the purgative effects of magnesia entirely depend on its meeting with an acid in the stomach, ... and as it will not produce scarcely any sensible

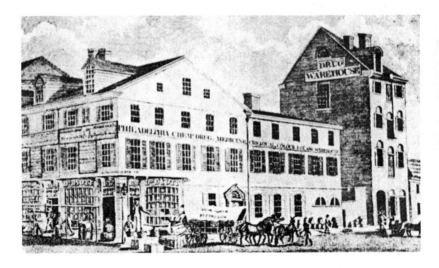

Fig. 43. Thomas Dyott operated, in 1807 in Philadelphia, one of the first drug warehouses which supported a national wholesale trade. This illustration (from Porter, T.: The Picture of Philadelphia, 1831) shows a Conestoga wagon being loaded with crates and barrels of drugs.

effect if an acid does not exist in the stomach, no reliance can be placed on it as a purgative."[9] Reece commented that "the magnesia sold in bottles at a most extravagant price, under the name of Henry's magnesia, is in no respect superior to the calcined magnesia of the Chemical Hall, 170 Piccadilly" (also the supplier of medical chests, Tables 16–17).

B. Multifarious Applications of Emetics

As will be documented below, emetics were highly valued in the physicians' materia medica during the early nineteenth century. Indeed, next to blood-letting, these agents were the most used in everyday practice in that era, a fact we can retrospectively ponder in dismay because 1) we now know their most popular emetic (tartar of antimony) is extremely toxic, and 2) only rarely is induced emesis of any medical value, and its induction in most diseases for which it was employed would be risk associated. The rationale for using emetics, as generally perceived in 1820, was summarized by Dr. William Sweetser, in *The New-England Journal of Medicine and Surgery*[10]:

> Besides the benefit arising from the evacuation of offensive matter often contained in the stomach, and this is by no means trifling, emetics are the most powerful means we possess of restoring to the inflamed parts their natural secretions, and promoting expectoration, which we know is here of the greatest importance. They aid also, to abate the inflammation by diminishing the action of the heart, and by their tendency to restore to the extreme vessels their natural functions. They also give a peculiar shock to the whole system, seeming to excite in it a new set of actions, to which in

many other affections much has been attributed; and although the benefit arising from this, may not be so great here as in fever, and some other diseases, still we may attribute to it some good. When an emetic is employed at the very onset of the disease, that is, within the first few hours of the attack, it is very generally sufficient to restore to the diseased parts their healthy actions, and thus we may often, without any other remedy, effect a perfect cure, or to say the least, we may in this way lay a foundation for the cure, the disease almost always being more manageable afterwards.

Dr. Chapman outlined the practical application of emetics.[2] His was the view, in opposition to Magendie, that the stomach was not passive, but active in the operation of vomiting (known today to be true). Chapman reported

it is remarkable, that whereas most other medicines lose their power by repetition, emetics increase the susceptibility of the stomach to their impression the oftener they are used, till at last the very sight of them will excite vomiting.

He considered that

when the vessels of the head are full, or there is much general plethora, the emetic should be preceded by the loss of blood ... (this) renders the vomiting safe, and more easy and effectual. By neglecting this admonition, many a life has been either endangered or sacrificed, by apoplexy or haemoptysis.

Further, Chapman recommended that "as a general rule, emetics should be given on an empty stomach, and in the morning, acting then with greater certainty, and less distress." This general premise for the use of emetics, as described by Chapman, can be seen to relate to the elimination of excessive, inflammatory fluid from the body rather than simply removal of gastric contents. While this principle conforms to that widely held in the early nineteenth century, and in particular to the teachings of Broussais, Chapman claimed that his doctrines, though analogous to those of the Parisian, M. Broussais, were held and taught by him years before the writings of Broussais. In Chapman's *Elements of Therapeutics and Materia Medica*,[2] the patho-physiology of inflammation and the rationale for use of emetics is extensively described.

Dr. Henry Jeffreys, a London surgeon, also summarized the basis for the use of tartar emetic in "local inflammations"[11];

For the last thirty years, to our knowledge, there is scarcely a form of inflammation, or indeed of febrile excitement, in which all ranks of the profession have not been in the habit of prescribing antimonials, and generally the tartrite, as a controller of vascular action.

It has been estimated that

in nine cases out of ten, where it is prescribed by modern practitioners (in 1821), it is with the view of *lessening the activity of the circulation*, whether that be by increasing the cutaneous and various other secretions, by causing nausea at the stomach, or by any direct sedative effect which it may have on the circulating organs.

The most common emetic, as in the case of the compound mentioned by Jeffreys, was tartar emetic, a combination of antimony with potassium tartrate. This antimonial also acted as a diaphoretic (sweat enhancing activity), an expectorant, a sedative, an irritant, and a cathartic, its actions depending upon the dose and route of administration. Smaller doses induced diaphoresis and expectoration, and it was administered by rubbing into the palm of hands, by intravenous injection, by oral ingestion after mixing with molasses or thick gruel, and in plasters. Some physicians, such as the well-known Professor William Cullen of Edinburgh (1712–1790) recommended massive doses of antimony,[12] though there were ebbs and tides in the practices and popularity, and of recommended doses of antimony. Dr. Alder was one who showed more restraint in the use of emetics than Cullen, who "made them by far too fashionable." Alder suggested that "when they do good (independently of clearing the stomach), it is by drawing the fluids from the internal to the external parts, and relaxing the skin so as to let them off. Also in inflammatory cases (not purely febrile) they do good by relaxing the inflammatory contraction of the arteries."[13] Other forms of this emetic also included sulphurated antimony, flowers of antimony (oxide of antimony), antimony iodide, and antimony trichloride. French and Italian physicians, especially Giovanni Rasori (1766–1826), were strong advocates of the use of tartar emetic. Rasori first employed tartar emetic in 1799 in the treatment of epidemic fever victims in Genoa, giving large doses, upwards to sixty grains per twenty-four hours.[12]

The numerous powers of emetic tartar were endorsed by Dr. William Balfour of London, in 1818 in a 92-page booklet entitled, *Observations, with cases, illustrative of the sedative and febrifuge powers of emetic tartar*.[14] These cases claimed beneficial effects in pneumonia, inflammatory gout, rheumatism (chronic and acute), cynanche tonsillaris, idiopathic fever, hernia humoralis, chronic inflammation of the bladder, etc. Also, a variety of "spasmodic" diseases were considered remedied by emetics, as outlined by Dr. Joseph Smith in a paper read before the Physico-Medical Society (London) in 1821.[15] These included spasmodic stricture of the urethra, producing retention of urine, puerperal convulsions, convulsions of children, tetanus, and in the spasmodic symptoms of hysteria and epilepsy. Emetics were recommended for the treatment of apoplexy by Tynicola[16] and Winterbottom,[17] in 1802 and 1803, respectively.

The efficacy of emetics was claimed by Rees in 1813 for treating hemoptysis, or the spitting of blood.[18] Different kinds of emetics were required, depending upon the degree of bleeding observed. "When the bleeding was very alarming, half a dram of sulph. zinci was given. When the bleeding was less urgent, one grain of tart. antimonii, to one scruple of ipecacuanha were given."

Tartarized antimony, administered by injection, was given for constipation, and ipecauanha was given for dysentery.[19] Cream of tartar (which sounds more like a sauce for fish) was given for respiratory distress[20] and pulmonary consumption in Ireland in 1808.[21] This (tuberculosis) was indeed an important disease to treat in this era, as Dr. Sharkey of Dublin commented that "it is a melancholy fact to state, that it appears by the London bills of mortality, that 40,000 persons die annually of pulmonary consumption within the city."[21]

Intravenous injection of dissolved emetic tartar (four grains) reportedly induced vomiting in a gentleman suffering from acute suffocation due to a piece of beef lodged in his throat, thereby saving his life in 1804.[22] Also, it allegedly counteracted salivation,[23] was used to treat stomachache (which was later shown by postmortem to be due to stomach cancer in a 52 year old woman).[24] Interestingly, emetics were also used in humans to treat poisonous snake bites, as described in 1803 by Dr. Benjamin Barton of Philadelphia.[25] Dr. Barton performed experiments on rabbits, dogs, and other animals subjected to snakebite, as he kept several captive rattlesnakes in his laboratory.

C. The Scourge of Venus and Mercury

The materia medica of the beginning of the nineteenth century included metallic compounds such as silver nitrate used for its astringent properties (for which it is still employed today) or for treatment of epilepsy,[26] [27] and the muriate of gold, for treatment of syphilis.[28] However, mercurial compounds were by far the most popular metallic compounds in use, particularly for syphilis. Because mercurial compounds are highly toxic to most biologic systems, the mercury-containing pharmaceuticals of the early nineteenth century elicited numerous toxic reactions; hence, the phrase describing these compounds as the "scourge of Venus and Mercury," when employed for treatment of venereal diseases was coined with satirical realism.

The widespread reliance upon mercurial compounds is exemplified by remarks, such as by Dr. Armstrong in 1818 and Dr. Robertson in 1824.

> Everyone knows how *much* under control are acute, and how *little* are chronic diseases! Want of general success in the *former* must be the Practitioner's own fault, provided he be early called in; for the united agency of blood-letting, purgatives, mercurials, blisters, and opium, will commonly subdue the very elements of the disorders, when judiciously and opportunely administered. We cannot say the same of chronic ailments.[29]

Though the modes of therapy have drastically changed, and the mechanisms of acute disorders have become greatly clarified in the late twentieth century, our current difficulty in understanding and treating *chronic* diseases (such as cardiovascular, and cerebrovascular disease and cancer) as compared to *acute* diseases remains a similar problem to today's clinicians! AttestTing to the effect of mercury on the living body, Robertson stated[30] in 1824 that

> the different preparations of mercury, particularly calomel, have of late years become of such general employment, not only in the hands of medical

Practitioners, but even as a domestic remedy, that there are but few diseases in which it is not most liberally administered; indeed, one would naturally conclude from its familiar use, that this remedy is at all times not only innocent in its effects, but that it is even a specific in the cure of the diseases for which it is given. But these are inferences which, by experience, I am far from admitting; and I am not only convinced that mercury is a remedy very precarious in its operation, but that it often is extremely pernicious in its effects.

Robertson was indeed sagacious in his comment about the pernicious effects of mercury, as this has been repeatedly confirmed in the late twentieth century, both in mammalian organisms and in the total ecosystem of animal, plant-environmental interactions.[31] Interestingly, the calomel referred to by Robertson, is an agent (mercurous chloride, which is partially converted in the intestine to more soluble mercuric ions) which was still used as a popular cathartic until recent years. It is now known that its cathartic action is uncertain, and that other laxatives are far more safe and effective. The inhibition by mercuric ions of enzyme systems (a common reaction to all heavy metals) results in the inhibition of active sodium transport from the intestinal lumen, retaining water and electrolytes in the gut which promotes catharsis by osmosis.

Some of the other forms of, and terms for mercury-containing compounds in use in the early nineteenth century were[2]:

hydrargyri nitrico-osydum: or *hydrargyrus nitratus ruber:*	"a red precipitate and sub-nitrate of Quicksilver, used as a powder or unguent, sprinkled on fungous or languid sores, to erode or stimulate."
hydrargyrum praecipitatum album: or *calix hydrargyri alba:*	"a white precipitate and ammoniated sub-muriate of mercury, mixed with lard for chronic eruptions."
hydrargyri oxymurias:	"a corrosive sublimite used for a lotion for venereal ulcers."
unguentum hydrargyri nitratis:	"citrine ointment, used for tinea capitis, tetter, etc., and for chronic inflammation of the tarsi, and reduced by mixture with lard or olive oil."
unguentum picis liquidae:	a tar ointment used in the above diseases. All of the above applications to be used "after the previous reduction of inflammation, by leeches, poultices, or other emollient means."

hydrargyrum cum Creta[32]:

preparations of mercury combined
with antimony and opium[32]:

acetate of mercury[33]:

confectio hydrargyri[34]:	mild preparation with molasses or manna.
pulvis hydrargyri[34]:	glychyrrhizae additive (also mild)
solutio hydrargyri[34]:	mild preparation with gum acacia and cinnamon

The above mercury compounds have also been reviewed in some detail in several early nineteenth century extensive treatises, including Dr. John Hamilton's 1819, *Observations on the Use and Abuse of Mercurial Medicines in Various Diseases*,[35] Dr. Henry Thomson's 1820, *An Inquiry into the Effects of Mercury on the Human Body, with a View to Estimate its Value as a Remedy in Several Important Diseases*,[36] and Dr. John's Bacot's 1821 volume,[37] *Observations on Syphilis, principally with References to the Use of Mercury in that Disease*. Hamilton declared

> that a medicine which, in one shape or other, is of such universal application as mercury, should be misused by ignorance, carelessness, or temerity, cannot be wondered at; but that these *abuses* should be blazoned forth as the common and general effects of the remedy, by clamorous terrorists, is somewhat derogatory to that cool, and chaste, and inductive philosophy, by which the present race is anxious to be distinguished.[35]

The toxic reactions to mercury were a subject of great dispute during the early decades in the nineteenth century. Dr. Davies commented:

> Although the current of abuse has run strongly against mercury in the writings of some modern reformers, and although there was some foundation for the reprehension of the abuses of this powerful medicine in the hands of ignorance and rashness; yet, among all sober-minded practitioners, the medicine holds its original rank, and is more depended on, in a great variety of diseases, than any other article of the pharmacopoeia.[34]

Dr. John W. Francis prepared his doctoral dissertation on quicksilver, in 1811, and included an analysis on its abuses.[38] One of the pathophysiologic responses observed after chronic mercury poisoning is ptyalism, or excessive secretion of saliva. This was commonly reported in the early nineteenth century. However, at that time ptyalism was considered to be a desirable effect by some physicians, though this was a disputed conclusion, as discussed by Wheaton of Rhode Island, in 1809.[39] Examples abound of this toxic side effect, such as those reported in the *Medico-Chirurgical Journal*: "Fifteen grains of calomel in conjunction with cathartics (was administered) in a threatening case of puerperal fever. The lady had nine copious stools, and yet in fifteen hours a smart ptyalism took place."[40] Sore mouth was also frequently seen as a toxic reaction. Cynanche laryngea, treated by tracheotomy and mercury, was followed seven days later by "very sore mouth with a good deal of ptyalism, but not the slightest uneasiness in the situation of the larynx."[41] Other toxic reactions to mercury were characterized by Carmichael in 1815 as, "mercurial phagedena, nodes, pains, erethismus mercurialis, hydrargyria, debility, coma, general dropsy (for the cure of which he strongly recommends nitrous acid conjoined with digitalis), and pulmonary affections."[42]

Among the multitude of other maladies treated with mercury were hydrophobia (rabies). Though this was frequently a fatal disease for the person bitten by a rabid animal, occasional victims survived. Mercury was one of the prescriptions for victims of the "canine madness." Moseley successfully treated a woman bitten by a rabid dog, with

> strong mercurial ointment copiously applied to the neck, throat, legs and thighs. She was ordered an ammoniacal julep containing camphor and valerian-root. In about 24 hours she began to be salivated. The next day, as the quicksilver purged her, its operation upon the intestines was restrained by the chalk-julep, cinnamon-water and and laudanum.[43]

Remarkably, she recovered. Mercury was also used experimentally by one Walter Trevelyan, Esq., who attempted to cure infected dogs of rabies, in 1806.

> Respecting the origin of canine madness in animals, after questioning the validity of the opinions which refer it to certain remote causes, as putrid ailment, climate, deficiency of water, want of perspiration, and lastly, what is called the *worm under the tongue*, (the opinion was offered) ... that the disease is never generated in animals but by contagion.

Trevelyan kept hounds for sporting, for many years, and

> during which time, I have not had less than fifty couples of them go mad; not a single one could I cure by any medicine that was administered. The Ormskirk remedy was given in doses innumerable; worming under the tongue was also found useless. Sea bathing, large bleedings, and mercury, exhibited in various forms and quantities, were all tried in vain.[44]

Hydrocephalus was treated with mercurials and diuretics without success,[45] as would be expected. Tumors of the tongue were cured in a woman "by use of the blue pills (mercury), and frictions, so as to produce considerable ptyalism...."[46] The following case history of recovery of a Scottish boy afflicted with tetanus following a lacerated wound, reported in 1810, also illustrates the alleged benefits of mercurial therapy:

A boy, 14 years of age, had his hand torn by a wheel. No material inconvenience was felt for ten days after the accident; he then began to complain of stiffness about his neck and chin; his jaw became locked; and this symptom was followed by pain at the sternum, spasmodic contraction of the abdominal muscles, and rigid contraction of all the muscles of his extremities and back; a quick and small pulse, and great anxiety in his countenance. The wound in his hand was not inflamed or painful, but went on healing, as if the system had not been at all deranged. Affusion of cold water was applied, without any relief to the symptoms; calomel and opium were administered internally, in large doses, for several days; but the disease kept increasing, though not in a violent degree. The warm bath was then ordered, and half an ounce of strong mercurial ointment was rubbed over the abdomen, and on the inside of the thighs and arms after coming from the bath, every night and morning. These remedies were carefully administered for four days, with manifest advantage. No salivation was produced by the mercury; and no apparent effect, except violent diarrhoea, which began on the second day after employing mercurial frictions; and this was allowed to continue unchecked for several days, as the most urgent symptoms gradually abated, while the bowels were so much relaxed. When the symptoms of tetanus had subsided, some restringent medicine was given; and at the end of three weeks from the commencement of the trismus, the boy was perfectly recovered.[47]

Consumption of the lungs (pulmonary tuberculosis), or phthisis pulmonalis, was treated, unsuccessfully, with calomel per os.[48] Two females (in 1811 and 1812) with "severe affections of the brain," such as irregular symptoms of hysteria (catamenia) and convulsions, or mania were treated by a course of mercurial friction, with reported full recovery.[49]

Fevers and dysenteries were treated with mercury, though the effectiveness of this agent was debated by early nineteenth century physicians. "It has been very erroneously considered that the free exhibition of mercury in fevers, dysenteries, and acute inflammations, is a new and dangerous practice, principally derived from the medical men of hot climates."[50] Dr. Abner Howe reported in the United States in 1819,

> As fever, in its various forms, destroys more of the human race, than any other disease, it demands the first and unwearied attention of every physician, that its nature may be better understood and its termination less frequently fatal. Sydemham affirms, that the various forms of fever constitute two thirds of the diseases of mankind, and that as large a proportion as eight of nine of all who die, are cut off by febrile diseases.
>
> Having had for a number of years, an opportunity of paying some attention to fever in its various changes and termination, I have drawn the following inferences from the observations of others, and my own experience:
>
> 1st. That idiopathic fever is a unit, and naturally admits of no division.
> 2nd. That its type or character principally depends upon the state of the system at the commencement of the fever.
> 3rd. That the preparations of mercury form the most efficacious means for the cure of this disease.[51]

Typhus was treated as well by mercurial agents. In Dr. Armstrong's work on typhus,

> an attempt was made to show that a combination of calomel and opium, after bleeding and purging, had a strong tendency to restore the balance between the venous and arterial systems, by rousing the heart into play, and thus removing acute and sudden congestions.[29]

One of Armstrong's cases of typhus, a woman with a "congestive form of typhus," was treated with calomel and jalap.

> In this lady, the liver seemed to be the principal seat of congestion, and partly on this account, and her extreme delicacy, the cure was chiefly confided to aperients and mercury; though the warm bath was occasionally used, and a moderate portion of diffusible stimulus allowed, whenever she felt faint from the evacuation.[51]

Another case of typhus was treated in 1808 in the United States:

> A delicate young lady in Philadelphia, in typhus, began with one tablespoonful of Madiera wine, and proceeded to two in a day, and before she was cured, consumed 127 bottles. Where mercury may be given, it is certainly better to try it, whether we consider economy, the rapidity effected in the cure, or the injury which the constitution is saved from, by cutting short an enervating and alarming disease.[52]

Yellow fever,[53] acute rheumatism,[54] liver disease,[35] affections of the stomach,[35] and even ophthalmia and impotence[55] were treated with mercurial medicines. Adverse effects on the heart were reported by Pearson, i.e., "in some instances, mercury affects the heart with partial, and in some cases with complete paralysis, the same as the extremities, and frequently produces sudden death."[56] Yet, of all the diseases treated with mercury, syphilis was the one malady for which this form of therapy was relatively unchallenged[33,40,42,57-59] at the dawn of the nineteenth century. Further, throughout the rest of that century and later, as the pathophysiology of disease became much more clarified, mercury remained a popular drug for this disease.

> The rage for novelty pervades ... (medicine) in common with others; there is a fashion even in medicine; and it would seem, that it matters not, however absurd and preposterous the opinions of some men are, so that they are but new and singular. —*Medical and Physical Journal* 19 (1808) 315.

Epilogue

In concluding a treatise documenting the status of medicine and physiology in the early nineteenth century, it is fitting to present a brief case history of the demise of one of America's greatest statesmen, General George Washington. This event, which occurred in 1799, was described by James Craik, Washington's attending physician, and Elisha C. Dick, a consulting physician, and was published for the benefit of the general public in *The Times*, a newspaper printed in Alexandria, Virginia and dated in December, 1799. Later these final medical attempts to save America's first president were republished in *The Philadelphia Medical Museum*, Volume 4, 154, 1808. This case history is noteworthy not only because of the patient's historic esteem, but as well because it captures the essence of early nineteenth century heroic therapy, including blood-letting, use of purgatives, application of blisters to the extremities, etc. Further, this case elicited a controversial dialogue between the British physician, John Reid, and the Americans who treated Washington, thus affording a typical example of the type of published debates in medical therapy in this era. Reid criticized the excessive blood-letting (80–90 ounces in twelve hours) of the debilitated General Washington by the American physicians, though condescending that "A British physician may be deemed not competent to ascertain the propriety of trans-atlantic practice; the current of blood, in the inhabitants of the new world, may bear some proportion to the current of its rivers...."[1]

It might be speculated that had Washington's therapy been undertaken in 1825 rather than in 1799, less copious blood-letting would have been employed by his attending physicians, but that the other therapeutic modes would have been the same, and the fatal outcome inevitable in any circumstance. The demise of this great American was presented, as follows:

> Some time in the night of Friday the 13th instant, having been exposed to rain on the preceding day, General Washington was attacked with an inflammatory affection of the upper part of the wind-pipe, called in technical language, *cynanche trachealis*. The disease commenced with a violent ague, accompanied with some pain in the upper and fore part of the throat, a sense of stricture in the same part, a cough, and a difficult rather than a painful deglutition, which were soon succeeded by fever and a quick and laborious respiration. The necessity of blood-letting suggesting itself to the

General, he procured a bleeder in the neighbourhood, who took from his arm, in the night, twelve or fourteen ounces of blood: he would not by any means be prevailed upon by the family to send for the attending physician till the following morning, who arrived at Mount Vernon at about eleven o'clock on Saturday. Discovering the case to be highly alarming, and foreseeing the fatal tendency of the disease, two consulting physicians were immediately sent for, who arrived, one at half after three, the other at four o'clock in the afternoon. In the interim were employed two copious bleedings; a blister was applied to the part affected, two moderate doses of calomel were given, and an injection was administered, which operated on the lower intestines—but all without any perceptible advantage; the respiration becoming still more difficult and distressing. Upon the arrival of the first of the consulting physicians, it was agreed, as there were yet no signs of accumulation in the bronchial vessels of the lungs, to try the result of another bleeding, when about thirty-two ounces of blood were drawn, without the smallest apparent alleviation of the disease. Vapours of vinegar and water were frequently inhaled, ten grains of calomel were given, succeeded by repeated doses of emetic tartar, amounting, in all, to five or six grains, with no other effect than a copious discharge from the bowels. The powers of life seemed now manifestly yielding to the force of the disorder. Blisters were applied to the extremities, together with a cataplasm of bran and vinegar to the throat. Speaking, which was painful from the beginning, now became almost impracticable; respiration grew more and more contracted and imperfect, till half after eleven o'clock on Saturday night, when, retaining the full possession of his intellect, he expired without a struggle.

He was fully impressed at the beginning of his complaint, as well as through every succeeding stage of it, that its conclusion would be mortal, submitting to the several exertions made for his recovery rather as a duty than from any expectation of their efficacy. He considered the operations of death upon his system as coeval with the disease; and several hours before his decease, after repeated efforts to be understood, succeeded in expressing a desire that he might be permitted to die without interruption.

During the short period of his illness he economized his time in the arrangement of such few concerns as required his attention, with the utmost serenity, and anticipated his approaching dissolution with every demonstration of that equanimity for which his whole life had been so uniformly and singularly conspicuous.[1]

[1]Craik, J. and E. C. Dick, On the death of General George Washington, The Philadelphia Medical Museum, 4 (1808) 154-156.

Chapter References

Chapter I

1. Palmer, R.R. *The World of the French Revolution*, Harper, New York, 1971, p. 79.
2. Hartwell, R.M. The rising standard of living in England, 1800-1850, *in* Black, E.C. (Ed.), *European Political History, 1815-1870, Aspects of Liberalism*, Harper and Row, Pub., New York, 1967, pp. 13-44.
3. Dampier, W.C. *A History of Science and its Relations with Philosophy and Religion*, 4th Ed., Cambridge Univ. Press, Cambridge, 1968, pp. XVI-XVII.
4. Duncan, A. Sr. and Duncan, A. Introduction to Volume 6. The Medical and Chirurgical Review 6 (1799) 1.
5. Coleman, W. *Biology in the Nineteenth Century: Problems of Form, Function, and Transformation*. Cambridge Univ. Press, London, 1977, pp. 1-167.
6. Magendie, F. *Précis élémentaire de physiologie*, 2 vols., Paris, 1816-1817.
7. Cuvier, G. *The Animal Kingdom Arranged According to its Organization*, Deterville, Paris, 1817.
8. Gardner, E.J. *History of Biology*, 3rd Ed., Burgess, Minneapolis, 1972, pp. 231-236.
9. Rothstein, W.G. *American Physicians in the Nineteenth Century*. The Johns Hopkins Univ. Press, Baltimore, 1972, pp. 1-230.
10. Tupper, Mr., Comment, Medical and Physical Journal 8 (1802) 500-504.
11. Buchan, W. *Domestic Medicine*, 22nd Ed., London, 1826, p. 98.

Chapter II

1. Kratzenstein, C.G. *Abhandlung über dem Nutzen Elektricität in der Arzneiswisschaft*, 2nd Edit., Halle, 1745.
2. Hartmann, J.F. *Die angewandte Electricität bei Krankheiten des menschlichen Körpers*, Hannover, 1770.
3. Deiman, J.R. *Geneeskundige proeven en waarnemingem omtrent de goede uitwerking der electriciteit*, Amsterdam, 1779.
4. Priestley, J. *Experiments and Observations on Different Kinds of Air*, 3 vols., London, 1774-1777.
5. Hackmann, W.D. The researches of Dr. Martinus Van Marum (1750-1837) on the influence of electricity on Animals and Plants. Med. History, 16 (1972) 11-26.
6. Wilkinson, C.H. *Elements of Galvanism in Theory and Practice*, 2 vols. Murray, London, 1804.
7. Editor. Historical statement of the Galvanic discovery, and of the publications that have appeared on that subject. Medical and Physical Journal, 7 (1802) 70-73.
8. Journal Correspondent at Paris. On the causes of irritability and excitability; by M. De La Melhere. Medical and Physical Journal 10 (1803) 25-29.
9. Van Barneveld, W. An account to imitate the effects of the torpedo by electricity. Philosophical Transactions of the Royal Society of London, 46 (1776) 196-225.

10. Editor. Article Number 17 pertaining to galvanism. The Medical and Chirurgical Review, 7 (1800) 314–315.

11. Pfaff, M. Refutation of the galvanic experiments of M. Von Humboldt. The London Medical Review and Magazine 6 (1801) 174–175.

12. Van Marum, M. On the theory of Franklin, according to which electrical phenomena are explained by a single fluid. Annals of Philosophy 26 (1820) 440–453.

13. Cuthbertson, J. Practical electricity, and galvanism, containing a series of experiments calculated for the use of those who are desirous of becoming acquainted with that branch of science; illustrated with nine copper plates. Medical and Physical Journal 20 (1808) 474–476.

14. Jones, Rev. W. Six letters on electricity. The London Medical Review 7 (1801) 415–426.

15. Bostock, J. Theory of the action of the galvanic apparatus. The Medical and Chirurgical Review 9 (1802) 275–279.

16. Editor. Comment of Mr. Carlisle and galvanism. The Medical and Chirurgical Review 7 (1800) 96.

17. Editor. Galvanism. The Medical and Chirurgical Review 6 (1800) 68–73.

18. Duncan, A. Sr. and Duncan, A. Jr. *Annals of Medicine for the Year 1798: Exhibiting a Concise View of the Latent and Most Important Discoveries in Medicine and Medical Philosophy*, Vol. 3, 556 pages, Mudie, Edinburgh, 1799. Reviewed in The Medical and Chirurgical Review 6 (1799–1800) 1–6.

19. Editor. Comment on Mr. Robertson and Galvanism. The Medical and Chirurgical Review 7 (1800) 483.

20. Editor. New discoveries in galvo-electricity. The Medical and Chirurgical Review 14 (1807) 94–98.

21. Editor. Difference between electricity and galvanism. The Medical and Chirurgical Review 14 (1807) 138.

22. Wilson, P. Identity of galvanism and the nervous influence vindicated. London Medical and Physical Journal 35 (1816) 423–424.

23. Wilson, P. Some observations relating to the agency of galvanism in the animal economy, in a letter addressed to the Editor of the Quarterly Journal of the Royal Institution. London Medical Repository, Monthly Journal and Review 12 (1820) 431–436.

24. Editor. Historical statement of the galvanic discovery, and of the publications that have appeared on that subject. Medical and Physical Journal 7 (1802) 159–161.

25. Wilkinson, C.H. *Elements of galvanism, in theory and practice; with a comprehensive view of its history, from the first experiments of Galvani to the present time. Containing, also, practical directions for constructing the galvanic apparatus, and plain systematic institution for performing all the various experiments*. 2 vols. Murray, London 1804. Reviewed in The Medical and Chirurgical Review 10 (1804) 364–376.

26. Hare, R. A new theory of galvanism, supported by some experiments and observations made by means of the calorimeter, a new galvanic instrument; also a new mode of decomposing potash extemporaneously. Annals of Philosophy 14 (1819) 176–184.

27. Grapengiesser. Observations and experiments, made with the view of employing galvanism for the cure of several diseases. Medical and Physical Journal 8 (1802) 315–324.

28. Wilson Philip, A.P. Some observations relating to the agency of galvanism in the animal economy, in a letter addressed to the Editor of the Quarterly Journal of the Royal Institution. The Quarterly Journal of Science, Literature, and the Arts 8 (1820) 72–83.

29. Editor. Comment by Berzelius on the distinction of positive and negative electricity. The Quarterly Journal of Science, Literature, and the Arts 17 (1824) 377.

30. Phillips, R. Electricity and galvanism explained on the mechanical theory of matter and motion. London Medical Repository, Monthly Journal and Review 14 (1820) 233–239.

31. Editor. Comments on galvanic electricity. The Medical and Chirurgical Review. 7 (1800) 293–295.

32. Van Marum, M. and Pfaff, M. Letter to Professor Volta, being an account of the results of some comparative experiments made with the Teylerian electrical apparatus

and Volta's metallic pile. (Abridged by Luke Howard). The Philosophical Magazine 12 (1803) 161-164.

33. Editor. Galvanism. The Philosophical Magazine 10 (1801) 93-95.

34. Hare, R. Letter to Prof. B. Silliman of Yale College — on some improved forms of the galvanic deflagrator — on the superiority of its deflagrating power: also, an account of an improved single leaf electrometer — etc. The Philadelphia Journal of the Medical and Physical Sciences 8 (1824) 118-125.

35. Hare, R. Letter description of an electrical plate machine, the plate mounted horizontally, and so as to show both negative and positive electricity. The Philadelphia Journal of the Medical and Physical Sciences 6 (1823) 104-106.

36. Editor. Comment on galvanism. The Medical and Chirurgical Review 8 (1801) 283-287.

37. Oersted, Prof. New electromagnetic experiments. Annals of Philosophy 16 (1820) 375-377.

38. Editor. Description of Mr. Davy's grand galvanic battery. Medical and Physical Journal 20 (1808) 254-255.

39. Editor. On the progress of galvanism. Medical and Physical Journal 6 (1801) 209-217.

40. Unnamed Correspondent (Letter to Editor). Experiments and Remarks on Galvanism. The Philosophical Magazine 9 (1800) 352-355.

41. Moyes, Dr. Letter to Dr. Garthshore, containing an account of some interesting experiments with M. Volta's galvanic pile. The Philosophical Magazine 9 (1800) 217-221.

42. Editor. Method of decomposing solution of arsenious acid by the galvanic pile. The Medico-Chirurgical Journal and Review 1 (1816) 452-453.

43. Editor. Facts and discoveries respecting galvanism. The London Medical Review 7 (1801) 462-464.

44. Guyton. Memoir on the theory of electricity. Medical and Physical Journal 8 (1802) 478.

45. Editor. Comments on galvanism and galvano-animal electricity. The Medical and Chirurgical Review 9 (1802) 498-500.

46. Editor. Memoires sur les causes de l'électricité. Journal de Chimie Médicale, de Pharmacie et de Toxicologie 1 (1825) 346-347.

47. Heidman, M.J.A. Some account of a new theory of galvanic electricity, founded on experiments. Medical and Physical Journal 28 (1807) 245-250.

48. Golding, B. Electricity. The Medico-Chirurgical Journal and Review 1 (1816) 176-177.

49. Aldini, J. An account of the late improvements in galvanism, with a series of curious and interesting experiments performed before the Commissioners of the French National Institute, and repeated lately in the anatomical theatres of London. The Medical and Chirurgical Review 10 (1803) 123-131.

50. Editor. On galvanism, and animal electricity. The Medical and Chirurgical Review 9 (1802) 576-577.

51. Editor. New galvanic apparatus. The London Medical Repository, Monthly Journal and Review 4 (1815) 344.

52. Editor. Animal magnetism. The Quarterly Journal of Science, Literature, and the Arts 9 (1820) 425.

53. Wilson Philip, A.P. An experimental inquiry into the laws of the vital functions, with some observations on the nature and treatment of internal diseases. The Medico-Chirurgical Journal 1 (1818-19) 394-399.

54. Editor. Galvanism. The Philosophical Magazine 11 (1802) 189-190.

55. Caldwell, M. Medical theses on galvanism. The Medical and Chirurgical Review 14 (1807) 125-129.

56. Home E. Hints on the subject of animal secretions. The Philosophical Magazine 35 (1810) 108-113.

57. Editor. Dr. Augustin, on the medical use of Galvanism. Medical and Physical Journal 7 (1802) 242-249.

58. Editor. Medical and Physical Intelligence; Notes on Galvanism. Medical and Physical Journal 11 (1804) 94-95.

59. Aldini, J. An account of the Galvanic experiments. Medical and Physical Journal 9 (1803) 382-385.

60. Editor. Medical and Physical Intelligence; Galvanism. Medical and Physical Journal 9 (1803) 195-196.

61. Mongiardini, A. On the application of galvanism in the cure of diseases. Medical and Physical Journal 17 (1807) 190.

62. Editor. Dr. Augustin, on the medical use of galvanism. Medical and Physical Journal 7 (1802) 242-249.

63. Grapengiesser, Dr. Observations and experiments made with an intention to employ galvanism in the cure of several diseases. Medical and Physical Journal 9 (1803) 131-153.

64. Editor. Mr. Strenger's use of galvanism. Medical and Physical Journal 9 (1803) 290-291.

65. Pfaff, M. On the effects of galvanism on the organ of hearing. The Medical and Chirurgical Review 9 (1802) 186.

66. Quensel, Dr. Galvanic experiments, applied to the uses of medicine. Medical and Physical Journal 8 (1802) 524-529.

67. Editor. Galvanism. The Philosophical Magazine 12 (1803) 374.

68. Whittam, J. Uber den Gebrauch des Galvanismus in der Epilepsie. Sommlung Auser. Abhand. zum Gebrausche pract. Aerzte 23 (1806) 630-634.

69. Whittam, J. Letter to Editors, On Epilepsy. Medical and Physical Journal 14 (1805) 527-528.

70. Mansford, J.G. *Researches into the Nature and Cause of Epilepsy, as connected with the Physiology of Animal Life, and Muscular Motion; with Cases illustrative of a new and successful Method of Treatment*, London, 1819, 162 pp. (Reviewed in The Medico-Chirurgical Journal 2 [1818-20] 216-220.)

71. Bardsley, S.A. Medical reports of cases and experiments, with observation; chiefly derived from hospital practice. The Medical and Chirurgical Review 15 (1807) 6-8.

72. Rademin, M. Mutisme de treize ans, gueri en neuf jours par le galvanisme. Bibliothèque Médicale 26 (1807) 123-124.

73. Wilkinson, C.H. *Elements of galvanism, in theory and practice; with a comprehensive view of its history, from the first experiments of Galvani to the present time; containing also, practical direction for constructing the galvanic apparatus, and plain systematic instructions for performing all the various experiments*. London, 1804, 468 pp. (Reviewed in Medical and Physical Journal 13 [1805] 82-87.)

74. Struve, Dr. Galvanodesme, ou moyen facile d'employer le Galvanisme dans les maladies nerveuses, dans l'asphyxie, et pour constater la mort. Bibliothèque Médicale 14 (1806) 255-257.

75. Cleaveland, P. Account of the effects of electricity. The New England Journal of Medicine and Surgery 2 (1813) 26-29.

76. Bally, V. Sur l'Emplie thérapeutique du galvanisme dans plasieures maladies. Revu Médicale Historique et Philosophique (Paris) 20 (1825) 41-58.

77. Teed, R. Experiment made with a galvanic belt, or chain. The Philosophical Magazine 12 (1803) 105-106.

78. Rossi, Prof. Efficacy of galvanism in cases of hydrophobia. Medical and Physical Journal 12 (1804) 259-262.

79. Waiblinger, Mr. Letter to editors on the effects of galvanism. Medical and Philosophical Journal 15 (1806) 150-153.

80. Golding, B. Electricity. Medico-Chirurgical Journal and Review 1 (1816) 362-4.

81. Editor. Account of the latest experiments on the application of galvanism, for medical purposes, made in Germany. Medical and Physical Journal 10 (1803) 330-334.

82. Bischoff, Dr. On galvanism and its medical applications. Medical and Physical Journal 7 (1802) 528-540.

83. Editor. Application of galvanism to the extraction of urinary calculi. The New England Journal of Medicine and Surgery 13 (1824) 219-220.

84. Hutchins, W. Galvanism. Medical and Physical Journal 9 (1803) 445-448.

Chapter III

1. Castiglioni, A. *A History of Medicine*. 2nd Ed., Alfred A. Knopf, N.Y. (1958) pp. 76-77, 174, 197, 380, 565.

2. Vaidy, J.F. On the efficacy of copious local bleeding in various complaints characterized by pain and spasm, as well as inflammation. The Medico-Chirurgical Journal 2 (1819-1820) 114-116.

3. Jackson, R. An outline of the history and cure of fever, endemic and contagious; more expressly the contagious fever of jails, ships, and hospitals; the concentrated endemic, vulgarly the yellow fever of the West Indies. The Medical and Chirurgical Review 6 (1799-1800) 317-330.

4. Rush, Dr. Essay on Gout, The Medical and Chirurgical Review 6 (1799-1800) 494.

5. Welsh, B. A practical treatise on the efficacy of blood-letting in the epidemic fever of Edinburgh. The Medico-Chirurgical Journal 2 (1819-1820) 278-281.

6. Mills, T. An essay on the utility of blood-letting in fever, illustrated by numerous cases; with some inquiry into the seat and nature of this disorder. The London Medical, Surgical, and Pharmaceutical Repository, Monthly Journal and Review 1 (1814) 424-425.

7. Vitet, M. *Of the Medicinal Leech*, The Medical and Physical Journal 26 (1811) 408-416.

8. Johnson, J.R. A treatise on the medicinal leech, including its medical and natural history, with a description of its anatomical structure: also, remarks upon the diseases, preservation, and management of leeches. The Medico-Chirurgical Journal 2 (1816) 481-496.

9. Norman, W. Case report no. VII on periodical affections. The Medico-Chirurgical Journal 2 (1819-1820) 141.

10. Ferguson, A. Letter to the editor. The Medical and Physical Journal 13 (1805) 299-303.

11. Dancer, T. Scriptures on Dr. Grant's Latin edition of his Essay on Yellow Fever. The Medical and Physical Journal 16 (1808) 413.

12. Beddoes, T. Researches, anatomical and practical, concerning fever as connected with inflammation. The London Medical Review 1 (1808) 283-294.

13. Editor. Gastro-entéro-colite avec phénomènes cérébraux. Annales de la Médecine Physiologique 1 (1822) 372-373.

14. Michelelant, Dr. Hernie Inguinale etranglée, guérée par les sangsues. Annales de la Médecine Physiologique 4 (1823) 145.

15. Dihmar, J. Notice sur les avantages des depletions sanguines dans la pluport des maladies. Annales de la Médecine Physiologique 4 (1823) 146-165.

16. X.Y. Cases of fever in children treated by leeches. The Medical and Physical Journal 31 (1814) 363-365.

17. Crampton, Dr. On the application of leeches to internal surfaces. The Medical Intelligencer 3 (1822) 396.

18. Kentish, Mr. A case of mortification of the toes and foot. The Medical and Chirurgical Review 6 (1799-1800) 48.

19. Yelloly, J. Observations on the vascular appearance in the human stomach, which is frequently mistaken for inflammation of that organ. The Medico-Chirurgical Transactions 4 (1819) 374-427.

20. Welsh, J. Description of a substitute for leeches. The London Medical and Physical Journal 34 (1815) 64.

21. Vaughan, Dr. An account of local inflammation and general disease following the operation of blood-letting. The Medical and Chirurgical Review 6 (1799-1800) 276.

22. Autenrieth, Dr. Easy method of stopping too violent bleedings after the application of leeches. The Medico-Chirurgical Journal and Review 2 (1816) 262-263.

23. Stuart, J. Observations on the occasional injurious effects of leeches. The Medical and Physical Journal 19 (1808) 57-60.

24. Wilkinson, G. Some remarks on the preservation and management of leeches. The Medical and Physical Journal 12 (1804) 485–496.

25. Ring, Mr. Letter to the editor. The Medical and Physical Journal 12 (1804) 357–358.

26. O'Berne, J.P. On the best mode of applying leeches. The London Medical and Physical Journal 35 (1816) 275.

27. S.M. On cutting off the tails of leeches. The London Medical and Physical Journal 35 (1816) 352.

28. Parker, Mr. Letter to the editor. The Medical and Physical Journal 14 (1805) 186.

29. Bishop, Mr. Letter to the editor. The Medical and Physical Journal 15 (1806) 198.

Chapter IV

1. Basalla, G. William Harvey and the heart as a pump. Bulletin of the History of Medicine 36 (1962) 467.

2. Parry, C.H. *An experimental inquiry into the nature, cause, and varieties of the arterial pulse; and into certain other properties of the larger arteries in animals, with warm blood, illustrated by engravings.* London, Underwood, 1816.

3. Kerr, G. *Observations on the Harveian Doctrine of the circulation of the blood.* pp. 100, London, 1816. Reviewed by A. Ewing. Medico-Chirurgical Journal 5 (1818) 392.

4. Carson, J. On the circulation of the blood in the head. The Journal of Foreign Medical Science and Literature 4 (1824) 409.

5. Bichat, X. *Anatomie Générale*, Reviewed in The London Medical Review 2 (1808–09) 67.

6. Shearman, W. Observations on the power of the arteries in carrying on the circulation of the blood, on the nature of this power, and on the manner of its exertion. The Journal of Foreign Medical Science and Literature 4 (1824) 1.

7. Editor. On the agents of the cirulation of the blood, in the arterial system. The New England Journal of Medicine and Surgery 2 (1813) 9–19.

8. Magendie, F. Mémoire sur l'action des artéres dans la circulation. J. de Physiol. Experiment. (Magendie) 1 (1821) 102–115.

9. Magendie, F. De l'influence des mouvements de la poctrine et des efforts sur la circulation du sang. J. de Physiol. Experiment. (Magendie) 1 (1821) 132–143.

10. Bell, C. *An Essay on the Forces which circulate the Blood; being an Examination of the Differences of the motions of Fluids in Living and Dead Vessels.* 83 pp. London, 1819, reviewed in Medico-Chirurgical Journal 2 (1819–20) 201–216.

11. Bell, C. A System of Dissections, explaining the Anatomy of the Human Body, the Manner of displaying the Parts, and their varieties in Disease. London, Johnson, 27 pp., 1798, reviewed in The Medical and Chirurgical Review 6 (1799–1800) 55–70.

12. Lucas, C.E. Observations on the relative powers of the heart and vessels in the support of the circulation of the blood. Medico-Chirurgical Review 1 (1820) 329–332.

13. Carson, J. *An Inquiry into the Causes of the Motion of the Blood, with an Appendix in which the Process of Respiration and its connection with the Circulation, are attempted to be elucidated.* London 1815, pp. 250, reviewed in The Eclectic Repertory and Analytical Review of Medicine and Philosophy 7 (1817) 368–390.

14. Hastings, C. Further observations and experiments on the motion of the blood. The London Medical Repository, Monthly Journal, and Review 8 (1817) 291–300.

15. Hastings, C. *A treatise on inflammation of the mucous membranes of the lungs, to which is prefixed, an experimental enquiry respecting the contractile power of the blood-vessels, and the nature of inflammation.* Underwoods, London, 1820, 420 pp. Reviewed in The London Medical and Physical Journal 44 (1820) 214–221.

16. Philip, A.P.W. Some observations relating to the power of circulation and the state of the vessels in an inflamed part. Medico-Chirurgical Transactions 12 (1823) 396–418.

17. Johnson, J. A reply to Mr. Hastings remarks on the circulation of the blood. The London Medical Repository, Monthly Journal, and Review 7 (1817) 364–375.

18. Fennel, W. Experiments and reflections on the cause of the vacuity of the arteries after death. Philadelphia Journal of the Medical and Physical Sciences 5 (1822) 68-75.

19. Joyce, Rev. J. *Letters on Natural and Experimental Philosophy, Chemistry, Anatomy, Physiology and Other Branches of Science Pertaining to the Material World.* J. Johnson & Co., London, 1810.

20. Editor. Philosophical transactions for 1809 (general science), New York Medical and Philosophical Journal and Review 2 (1810) 205-222.

21. Brickell, J. Sketches relative to the natural history of the blood, and a theory of gout. Medical Repository 6 (1808) 45-52.

22. Alderson, J. On the motion of the heart. The Quarterly Journal of Science, Literature, and the Arts 18 (1825) 223-228.

23. Nicholl, W. Primary elements of disordered circulation of the blood. The London Medical Repository, Monthly Journal, and Review 7 (1817) 441-449.

24. Mayer, M. On the absorbent power of the veins. The London Medical Repository, Monthly Journal and Review 10 (1818) 236-239.

25. Lawrence, O'B. Account of some further experiments to determine the absorbing power of the veins and lymphatics. The London Medical Repository, Monthly Journal, and Review 19 (1823) 516-520.

26. Home, E. Experiments to prove that fluids pass directly from the stomach to the circulation of the blood, and from thence into the cells of the spleen, the gall bladder, and urinary bladder, without going through the thoracic duct. The Eclectic Repertory and Analytical Review of Medicine and Philosophy 2 (1812) 160-165.

27. Harlan, R. Two experiments performed on living animals, to prove that the circulation of the blood, through the lungs, is immediately and entirely suppressed during expiration. The Eclectic Repertory and Analytical Review of Medicine and Philosophy 9 (1819) 122-128.

28. Sarlandiere, M. Memoire sur la circoulation du sang, éclairée par la physiologie et la pathologie, lu a l'académie royale des sciences. Annales de la Médicine Physiologique (Broussais) 1 (1822) 133-192.

29. Spallanzani, A. Experiments upon the circulation of the blood, throughout the vascular system: on languid circulation: on the motion of the blood, independent of the heart: and on the pulsations of the arteries (English Translation; Ridgway, London, 424 pp. 1801). Reviewed in The London Medical Review 8 (1802) 14-23.

30. Philip, A.P.W. Some observations on inflammation. The London Medical Repository, Monthly Journal, and Review 6 (1816) 51-57.

31. Editor. Critical analysis of experiments by Mr. Howship, London Medical and Physical Journal 36 (1816) 158-160.

32. Hodgson, J. *A Treatise on the Diseases of Arteries and Veins, Containing the Pathology and Treatment of Aneurisms and Wounded Arteries.* London, T. Underwood, 1815.

33. Dr. Baldwin. On two cases of diseased heart. The Philadelphia Medical Museum 5 (1808) 100-102.

34. Bourdon, I. Note sur l'Aphoniequi survient dans l'aneurysme de l'aorte. Revue Medicale (Historique et Philosophique) Paris 7 (1822) 57-60.

35. Nicoll, A. Account of a case of aneurism of the femoral arteries of both thighs, which occurred in a native of Travancore. The London Medical Repository Monthly Journal and Review 3 (1815) 371-374.

36. Dr. Neuman. Du rapport qu'il y a entre les grands et les petits vaisseaux sanguins, et de la nature de l'inflammation. Bibliothèque Medicale 24 (1806) 124-129, 260-266.

37. Dr. Vialle. On the circulation and excitement. Medico-Chirurgical Review 1 (1818-1819) 103-112.

38. Pinkerton, J.H.M. Kergaradec, friend of Laennec and pioneer of foetal auscultation. Proceedings of the Royal Society of Medicine 62 (1969) 477.

39. Mann, R.J. Scarpa, Hodgson, and Hope, artists of the heart and great vessels. Mayo Clinic Proceedings 49 (1974) 889.

40. Hodgson, J. *A treatise on the diseases of arteries and veins, containing the pathology and treatment of aneurisms and wounded arteries.* T. Underwood, London 1815.

41. Hale, E. *Experiments and observations on the communication between the stomach and the urinary organs, and on the propriety of administering medicine by injection into the veins.* (Boylston medical prize dissertations for the years 1819 and 1821). Oliver Everett and Joseph Ingraham, Boston 1821. Reviewed in The New England Journal of Medicine and Surgery 11 (1822) 163.

42. Ficarra, B.J. The evolution of blood transfusion. Ann. Med. Hist. 4 (1942) 302-323.

43. Leacock, J.H. On the transfusion of blood in extreme cases of haemorrhage. The Medico-Chirurgical J. and Rev. 3 (1817) 276-284.

44. Editor. The Family Oracle of Health, Economy, Medicine, and Good Living 1 (1824) 312-316.

45. Brande, W.T. Chemical researches on the blood, and some other animal fluids. The Eclectic Repertory and Analytical Review of Medicine and Philosophy 3 (1813) 293-306.

46. Bellingeri, Dr. The state of the blood, with regard to its electric phenomena. The J. Foreign Med. Sci. and Lit. 4 (1824) 583-585.

47. Editor. On the cause of the red colour of the blood. New York Medical and Philosophical Journal and Review 3 (1811) 300-301.

48. Berzelius, Dr. Colouring matter of the blood. The New England Journal of Medicine and Surgery 6 (1817) 407-408.

49. Parkinson, J. *The Chemical Pocket-book, or, Memoranda Chemica: arranged in a Compendium of Chemistry; with Tables of Attractions, calculated as well for the occasional Reference of the professional Student, as to supply others with a general knowledge of Chemistry.* 2nd Ed., with the latest Discoveries, Symonds, London, 1801, 250 pp., reviewed in London Medical Review 6 (1801) 113-115.

50. Hewson, T.T. Some experiments on the coagulation of the blood when out of the body. The Eclectic Repertory and Analytical Review of Medicine and Philosophy 1 (1811) 230-233.

51. Belhomme, M. Of the coagulation of the blood. The London Medical Repository, Monthly Journal and Review (new series) 2 (1824) 73-75.

Chapter V

1. Cartwright, F.F. The impact of infectious diseases (Chapter 5) in *Disease and History*, pp. 113-136, Thomas Y. Crowell Co., N.Y., 1972.

2. Melvyn Howe, G. *Man, Environment and Disease in Britain*, pp. 142-159, Barnes & Noble Books, N.Y., 1972.

3. Blane, Sir G., A statement of facts tending to establish an estimate of the true value and present state of vaccination, Medico-Chirurgical Trans. 10 (1819) 315-338.

4. Jenner, E., May 6, 1801, letter to editor. Medical and Physical Journal 5 (1801) 505-507.

5. Wachsel, J.C. Vaccination report from Hospital for the Small-pox, for Inoculation and for Vaccination, at Pancras, London Medical Repository and Monthly Journal and Review 11 (1819) 257.

6. Blane, Sir G. Comments on vaccination, The Eclectic Repertory and Analytical Review of Medicine and Philosophy 10 (1820) 297-311.

7. Pepys, L. April 10, 1807 Report of the Royal College of Physicians of London, on Vaccination. The Medical and Physical Journal 18 (1807) 97-111.

8. Moore, J. *The History and Practice of Vaccination*—a review thereof, The Eclectic Repertory and Analytical Review of Medicine and Philosophy 8 (1818) 522-538.

9. Blane, Sir. G. and E. Jenner. Selected comments on the value of vaccination. Medico-Chirurgical Review 1 (1820) 718-725.

10. Rush, B. An account of a case of small-pox after variolus inoculation. The Philadelphia Medical Musuem 5 (1808) 183-185.

11. Gillepsie, J.D. Report on cow-pox, Medical Repository 1 (1809) 87-90.

12. Halford, H. Farquhar, W., Heberden, W., Bree, R. and J. Hewey. Reports of

the National Vaccine Establishment, taken from the August, 1811 Philosophical Magazine. The Eclectic Repertory and Analytical Review of Medicine and Philosophy 2 (1812) 291–302.

13. Ring, J. Case of smallpox, twice after vaccination. The London Medical Repository, Monthly Journal and Review 3 (1815) 204–205.

14. Editor. Smallpox after vaccination — a case report. The London Medical Repository, Monthly Journal and Review 5 (1816) 295–296.

15. Millington. A case of natural smallpox, occurring several years after inoculation with various matter; in consequence of the progress of the inoculated pustules being interrupted. London Medical and Physical Journal 35 (1816) 477–478.

16. Editor. Comments on vaccination in Germany, Medical and Physical Journal 6 (1801) 571–572.

17. Editor. Comments on a conscious view of circumstances and proceedings respecting vaccine inoculation, London Medical Review 5 (1800–01) 157–160.

18. Ring, J. On vaccination, Medical and Physical Journal 18 (1807) 139–152.

19. Akerly, S. July 10, 1809 letter to Dr. Miller on practical remarks on vaccination as a preventative of small-pox, Medical Repository 2 (1810) 30–31.

20. Editor. Reprint from January 1810 Edinburgh Review, entitled, Report of the Royal College of Physicians of London on vaccination; with an appendix, containing the opinions of the Royal Colleges of Physicians of Edinburgh and Dublin, and of the Royal Colleges of Surgeons of London, of Dublin, and of Edinburgh. The Eclectic Repertory and Analytical Review of Medicine and Philosophy 1 (1811) 55–84.

21. Krauss, G.F. Die Shutzpockenimpfung, etc; ou de l'Inoculation de la Vaccine, Review Medicale (Historique et Philosophique) Paris 2 (1820) 65–81.

22. Editor. September 18, 1818 report in London Times, on vaccination in India, The Eclectic Repertory and Analytical Review of Medicine and Philosophy 9 (1819) 129–131.

23. Waterhouse, B. *The Rise, Progress and Present State of Medicine*, Boston, Fleet, 1792, p. 30.

24. Waterhouse, B. *A Project for Exterminating the Small-pox, Being the History of the Variolae Vaccinae or Kine-pox Commonly Called the Cow-pox As It Has Appeared in England. With an Account of a Series of Inoculations Performed for the Kine-Pox in Massachusetts*. Cambridge, Mass., W. Hilliard, 1800, 40 pp.

25. Waterhouse, B. *A Prospect for Exterminating the Small-Pox: II A Continuation of Narrative of Facts Concerning the Progress of the New Inoculation in America. Practical Observations in Local Appearance, Symptoms, and Treatment of Variola Vaccina or Kine Pock*. Cambridge, Mass., W. Hilliard, 1802.

26. Bloch, H., Benjamin Waterhouse (1754–1846), The Nation's First Vaccinator. Am. J. Dis. Child. 127 (1974) 226–229.

27. Walker. Annual Report of the London Vaccine Institution. The London Medical Repository, Monthly Journal and Review 5 (1816) 437.

28. Editor. Vaccination Society Report. The Eclectic Repertory and Analytical Review of Medicine and Philosophy 7 (1817) 122.

29. Editor. Vaccination report for the Small-pox Hospital, London, The Philadephia Medical Museum 1 (1805) 340.

30. Gregory, G. Cursory remarks on small-pox, as it occurs subsequent to vaccination. Medico-Chirurgical Transactions 12 (1823) 324–343.

31. Fermor, W., and E. Jenner. September letters, 1801 On Vaccination. Medical and Physical Journal 6 (1801) 323–343.

32. Editor. New Test for Vaccination, Medical Repository 1 (1809) 207–208.

33. Editor. Abstract of a Case of Vaccine, of uncommon magnitude. The Philadelphia Medical Museum 1 (1805) 305–307.

34. Hoare, J. Letter pertaining to vaccination, London Medical and Physical Journal 36 (1816) 9–10.

35. Editor. Vaccine inoculation, The Philosophical Magazine 12 (1803) 96.

36. Editor. Vaccine inoculation undertaken by Dr. Sacco of Milan. The Philosophical Magazine 12 (1803) 184–186.

37. Bryce, J. Review of book, *Practical Observations on the Inoculation of Cow Pox, Pointing*

Out a Test of a Constitutional Affection in Those Cases in which the Local Inflammation is Slight, and in Which the Fever is Perceptible, Edinburgh 1802, 236 pp., Medical and Physical Journal 8 (1802) 373–376.

38. Editor. Extract of a letter from Dr. De Carro of Vienna, on inoculation for the vaccine and the plague. The Philosophical Magazine 17 (1803) 288.

39. Editor. Account of Dr. M. Valli and vaccination for the plague. The Philadelphia Medical Museum 1 (1805) 342–344.

40. Archer, J. The hooping-cough cured by vaccination. Medical Repository 6 (1808) 182–183.

41. Cooke, T. Observations on some effects of vaccination on the constitution. The London Medical Repository, Monthly Journal and Review 3 (1815) 287–289.

42. Shearman, W. On vaccination. The London Medical Repository, Monthly Journal and Review 3 (1825) 113–119.

43. Editor. On the antiquity of the cow-pock, and of its inoculation time immemorial in Germany. The Philosophical Magazine 13 (1803) 395–399.

44. Editor. Extract of a January 21, 1801 letter from Dr. Marshall in Malta. The Philosophical Magazine 9 (1800) 187–191.

45. Editor. Extract of a February 14, 1801 letter from Dr. De Carro of Vienna to Dr. E. Jenner, Medical and Physical Journal 5 (1801) 351–352.

46. Editor. Vaccine inoculation, The Philosophical Magazine 12 (1803) 373–374.

47. Editor. Extracts from letters on vaccination by Christie, Jones and Ring, The Philadelphia Medical Museum 4 (1808) 134–192.

48. Editor. Report on the progression of vaccination, The London Medical Repository, Monthly Journal and Review 3 (1815) 36–41.

49. Editor. Reviews of the monographs, *The History and Practice of Vaccination,* London, 1817, 300 pp. (by J. Moore) and on *Account of an Epidemic Small Pox, which occurred in Cupar in Fife, in the Spring of 1817; and the Degree of protecting Influence which Vaccination afforded; accompanied with Practical Inferences and Observations,* Edinburgh, 1817, 38 pp. (by H. Dewar), Medico-Chirurgical Journal 5 (1818) 283–293.

Chapter VI

1. Linton, D. *The Bicentennial Almanac,* Thomas Nelson Inc., Pub., New York, 1975.

2. U.S. Bureau of the Census. *Historical Statistics of the United States, 1789–1945* (Washington: Government Printing Office, 1949, p. 25.)

3. White, D. *The Jeffersonians. A Study in Administrative History, 1801–1829.* The Free Press, New York. 1951.

4. Editor. Mortality Tables, The Electric Repertory and Analytical Review, Medical and Philosophical 10 (1820) 278–290.

5. Annual Reports from City Boards of Health, The Philadelphia Journal of the Medical and Physical Sciences 8 (1824) 238–249.

6. Thurston, J. Bill of mortality for Portsmouth, New Hampshire, for A.D. 1818. London Medical Repository, Monthly Journal, and Review 12 (1820) 261.

7. Major, R.H. *A History of Medicine,* Vol. 2, Charles C. Thomas, Springfield, 1954.

8. Valle, R.K. The Cesarean Operation in Alta California during The Franciscan Mission Period (1769–1833). Bull. Hist. Med. 48 (1974) 265–275.

9. Bell, W.J. Jr. Medical Practice in Colonial America, Bull. Hist. Med. 31 (1957) 442–453.

10. Sigerist, H.E. *American Medicine,* New York, Norton 1934, p. 3.

11. Bloch, H. Colonial Medicine. Its roots and background, N.Y. St. J. Med. 72 (1972) 2566–2568.

12. Knowles, J.H. The Struggle to Stay Healthy, Time Mag., Aug. 9, 32–34, 1976.

13. Packard, F.R. *History of Medicine in United States,* New York, Hafner, 1963.

14. Blake, J.B. Diseases and medical practice in colonial America, in *History of American Medicine, A Symposium,* New York, MD Publication, 1958.

15. Smith, W. *The History of the Province of New York ... to the Year MDCCXXXII* (London, 1757) p. 212. as cited in Bell, W.J. Jr., Medical practice in colonial America, Bull. Hist. Med. 31 (1957) 442–453.

16. Akerly, S. Account of the ergot or spurred rye, as employed in certain cases of difficult parturition. Med. Repos. 6 (1808) 341–347.

17. Hall, C.R. Jefferson on the medical theory and practice of his day, Bull. Hist. Med. 31 (1957) 235–245.

18. Shafer, H.B. *The American Medical Profession 1783–1850.* New York, Columbia University Press, 1936.

19. Rothstein, G. *American Physicians in the Nineteenth Century.* Baltimore, The Johns Hopkins University Press, 1972, pp. 125–151.

20. Thomson, S. *New Guide to Health: or Botanic Family Physician,* 3rd ed. Boston 1832.

21. Carter, R. "Remedies of Dr. Richard Carter of Kentucky" — 1825. From *A Short Sketch of the Author's Life, and Adventures from His Youth until 1818,* in the First Part. In Part II: "A Valuable, Vegetable, Medical Prescription, with Table of Detergent and Corroborant Medicines to Suit the Treatment of the Different Certificates." Published at Versailles, Indiana, 1825.

22. Berman, A. The Thomsonian Movement and its relation to American pharmacy and medicine. Bull. Hist. Med. 25 (1951) 405–428, 519–538.

23. Smith, J. A lecture on medical philosophy. New York Med. and Phys. J. 7 (1828) 168, 185, 174.

24. Daniels, G.H., Jr. Finalism and positivism in nineteenth century American physiological thought, Bull. Hist. Med. 38 (1964) 343–363.

25. Osler, W. Influence of Louis on American Medicine, Bull. The Johns Hopkins Hosp. 8 (1897) 161–167.

26. Mann, J. *Medical Sketches of the Campaigns of 1812, 13, 14* Dedham (Mass.) 1816.

27. Thacher, J. *A Military Journal during the American Revolutionary War,* Boston, 1823.

28. Ramsay, D. *Review of the Improvements, Progress and State of Medicine in the XVIIIth Century,* Charleston, 1801.

29. Bartlett, J. *A Dissertation on the Progress of Medical Science in the Commonwealth of Massachusetts,* Boston, 1810.

30. Thacher, J. *American Medical Biography, 2 vols.* Boston, 1825.

31. McDaniel, W.G. A view of the 19th century medical historiography in the United States of America, Bull. Hist. Med. 33 (1959) 415–435.

32. Waring, J.I. The Influence of Benjamin Rush on the practice of bleeding in South Carolina, Bull. Med. Hist. 35 (1961) 230–237.

33. Alexander, F.G. and S.T. Selesnick. *The History of Psychiatry,* Harper and Row, New York, 1966, pp. 106–132.

34. Duffy, J. Smallpox and the Indians in the American Colonies, Bull. Med. Hist. 25 (1951) 324–341.

35. Wright, R.D., Dr. Franklin. Pub. Hlth. Rep. 91 (1976) 178–183.

36. Rhodes, N.H. Evidence of the precise date of the cowpox in America, Phil. Mag. 16 (1803) 252–253.

37. Italia, S.R., Elisha North: Experimentalist, epidemiologist, physician, 1771–1834, Bull. Hist. Med. 31 (1957) 505–536.

38. Miller, E. Vaccine pox. Medical Repository 4 (1801) 321.

39. Waring, J.I. Charleston medicine 1800–1860, J. Hist. Med. Allied Sci. 31 (1976) 320–342.

40. Rothstein, W.G. *American Physicians in the Nineteenth Century.* Chapters 5–6, 1972, Baltimore, Johns Hopkins Univ. Press, pp. 85–121.

41. Briegar, G.H. (editor). *Medical America in the Nineteenth Century,* Chapter I; 1972, Baltimore, Johns Hopkins Univ. Press, pp. 3 –38.

42. Garland, J. The New England Journal of Medicine, 1812–1968, J. Hist. Med. 24 (1969) 125–139.

43. Drake, D., p. ix, cited in Reference 50, pp. 86–87. *Practical Essays on Medical Educations and the Medical Profession in the United States.*

44. Coventry, C.B. History of medical legislation in the State of New York, N.Y.J. Med. 4 (1845) 151-161.

45. Stanford, E. History of the laws regulating the practice of medicine, etc. in Louisiana, 1808-1878. New Orleans Med. and Surg. J. 5 (1878) 909-926.

46. Kett, J.F. American and Canadian medical institutions, 1800-1870, J. Hist. Med. Allied. Sci. 22 (1967) 343-356.

47. Norwood, W.F. *Medical Education in the United States before the Civil War*, Univ. Penn. Press, Philadelphia, 1944.

48. Fulton, J.F. Science in American universities 1636-1946, with particular reference to Harvard and Yale, Bull. Hist. Med. 20 (1946) 97-111.

49. Editor. Some account of Harvard University, in Cambridge, Massachusetts, New Eng. J. Med. Surg. 5 (1816) 109-126.

50. Klickstein, H.S. A Short history of the professorship of chemistry of the University of Pennsylvania School of Medicine 1765-1847 Bull. Hist. Med. 27 (1953) 43-68.

51. Moore, T.E., Jr. The early years of the Harvard Medical School—Its founding and curriculum, 1782-1810. Bull. Hist. Med. 27 (1953) 530-561.

52. Billings, J.S. Literature and Institutions, in E.H. Clarke, et al. A Century of American Medicine, Lea, Philadelphia, 1876, p. 359.

Chapter VII

1. Atkinson, J. Remarks on Dr. Kinglake's observations on the obstetric practice. London Medical & Physical Journal 36 (1816) 3.

2. Ramsbotham, J. *Practical Observations in Midwifery; with a Selection of Cases, Part 1.* London, 422 pp., 1821, reviewed in Medico-Chirurgical Review 2 (1821-22) 141 and Medical Repository 7 (1822) 162.

3. Merriman, S. On the art of midwifery, as exercised by medical practitioners, in reply to Dr. Kinglake. London Medical & Physical Journal 35 (1816) 282.

4. Arthure, H. The midwife-in Simpson's time and ours. J. Obstet. Gyn. Brit. Comm. 80 (1973) 1.

5. Schweighoeuser, J.F. Archives de l'Art des Accoucheurs, considéré sous ses Rapports anatomique, physiologique, et pathologique. Part 1, 187 pp., Strasbourg, 1801.

6. Kinglake, Dr. Kinglake in reply to Mr. Wayte and others, on obstetric practice. London Medical & Physical Journal 36 (1816) 2.

7. Power, J. *A Treatise of Midwifery; Developing new Principles, which tend materially to lessen the sufferings of the patient, and shorten the Duration of Labour.* 270 pp., London 1819, (Reviewed in Medico-Chirurgical Journal 2 (1819-20) 221.

8. Wayte, J. Remarks on Dr. Kinglake's opinions concerning the obstetric Art. London Medical & Physical Journal 35 (1816) 359.

9. Dewees, W.P. *A Compendious System of Midwifery, chiefly designed to facilitate the Inquiries of those who may be pursuing this Branch of Study*, illustrated by occasional Cases; with thirteen Engravings. 608 pp., Philadelphia (H.C. Carey and I. Lea) 1824 (Reviewed in The Phil. J. Med. Phys. Sci. 9 [1824] 168).

10, Dewees, W.P. *Essays on various subjects connected with Midwifery.* 480 pp. (Carey & Lea), Philadelphia, 1823. Reviewed in Medical Repository 8 (1824) 362.

11. Wales, T. On the necessity and importance of the accoucheur's profession. London Medical and Physical Journal 40 (1818) 17.

12. Delisle. A case of extra-uterine pregnancy, terminating in the extraction of a living child by an incision of the vagina. Bull Soc. Med. d'Emul., May & June, 1818. Reviewed in London Medical Repository, Monthly Journal and Review 10 (1818) 338.

13. Spalding, L. A singular case in midwifery. The Philadelphia Medical Museum 4 (1808) 51.

14. Joyce, J. (Rev.) *Letters on Natural and Experimental Philosophy, Chemistry, Anatomy, Physiology, and Other Branches of Science Pertaining to the Material World.* J. Johnson & Co., London pp. 368-381, 1810.

15. Michel, W. Essay on the causes which demand the Caesarian operation, read by appointment, before the Medical Society of South Carolina. The Carolina Journal of Medical Science and Agriculture 1 (1825) 248.

16. Burns, J. *The Principle of Midwifery; including the Diseases of Women and Children.* 5th Ed., London, 1820. (Reviewed in Medico-Chirurgical Review 1 [1820] 595.)

17. Conquest, J.T. Outlines of Midwifery, developing its Principles and Practice; with Twelve Lithographic Engravings. London, 193 pp., 1820. (Reviewed in Medico-Chirurgical Review 2 [1821–22] 47).

18. Akerly, S. Account of the ergot or spurred rye, as employed in certain cases of difficult parturition. Medical Repository 6 (1808) 341.

19. Saillant, in *Duncan's Medical Commentaries*, Vol. 5, p. 50, Philadelphia, 1795.

20. Editor. Section VII, Midwifery, The J. Foreign Medical Science and Literature 4 (1824) 215.

21. Clarke, J. On the effects of certain articles of food, especially oysters, on women after childbirth. Medical Transactions 5 (1815) 109.

22. Burns, J. The Principles of Midwifery; including the Diseases of Women and Children, Glasgow and London, 519 pp., 1809 (Reviewed in The Eclectic Repertory and Analytical Review of Medicine and Philosophy 1 [1811] 220; see also ref. 16).

23. Adams, J. On midwives and accoucheurs, London Medical and Physical Journal 35 (1816) 84–88.

24. Smellie, W. *A Set of Anatomical Tables, with Explanations, and an Abridgment of the Practice of Midwifery; with a View to Illustrate a Treatise on That Subject, and Collection of Cases*, Edinburgh, William Creech, 1792.

Chapter VIII

1. Editors. Reviews on monographs on peritoneal inflammation, by F.J.V. Broussais, M. Gasc, A. Abercrombie, C.R. Pemberton, and M. Montfalcon. Medico-Chirurgical Review 1 (1820) 161.

2. Fodera, M.A. An examination of some medical doctrines, compared with those of Dr. Broussais. Paris 1821, reviewed in Philadelphia Journal of the Medical and Physical Sciences 6 (1823) 35.

3. Miller, E. Some remarks on the importance of the stomach as a centre of association, a seat of morbid derangement, and a medium of the operation of remedies in malignant diseases. Medical Repository 5 (1802) 300.

4. Sutton, T. Considerations regarding pulmonary consumption. Medical and Physical Journal 6 (1801) 89.

5. Lespagnol, M. On cerebral inflammations as determined by affections of the digestive organs. Medico-Chirurgical Journal 3 (1817) 262.

6. Editor. Analytical report on contagion. Medico-Chirurgical Review 1 (1824) 50.

7. Cope, Sir Z. The growth of knowledge of acute abdominal diseases 1800–1900. Proceedings of the Royal Society of Medicine 57 (1964) 129.

8. Von Haller, A. *First Lines of Physiology*, Translated into English from the 3rd Latin Edition, Ed. 1 (American), Troy, N.Y., Obadiah Penniman and Co. 1803, pp. 317–318.

9. Vanderschilt, J.A. Dissertation sur la gastrite ou inflammation de l'estomac. Journal de Médecine, Chirurgie, Pharmacie etc. 36 (1816) 298.

10. Villeneuve, A.C.L. Observation pour servir a l'histoire du diagnostic des affections organiques de l'estomac. Journal de Médecine, Chirurgie, Pharmacie, etc. 34 (1815) 115.

11. Richond, L.J.R.A. De l'influence de l'estomac sur la production de l'apoplexie, d'après les principes de la nouvelle doctrine physiologique. Revue Médicale Historique et Philosophique (Paris) 15 (1824) 152.

12. Yelloly, J. Observations on the vascular appearance in the human stomach, which is frequently mistaken for inflammation of that organ. The Eclectic Repertory and Analytical Review 5 (1815) 1.

13. Pfeiffer, C.J. and Sethbhakdi, S. Vascular impairment—An etiologic factor in peptic ulcer disease? in *Peptic Ulcer*, C.J. Pfeiffer (editor) J.B. Lippincott, Philadelphia, 1971.

14. Cheyne, J. A case of melaena; with observations on the alternate excess of morbid action in the mucous and serous membranes. The Dublin Hospital Reports and Commentary in Medicine and Surgery 1 (1818) 259.

15. Cathrall, I. Memoir on the analysis of the black-vomit, ejected in the last stage of the yellow fever. London Medical Review 6 (1801) 204.

16. Roques, B. Observations sur la guérison d'une plaie pénétrante de l'abdomen, compliquée d l'ouverture de l'estomac et de l'arc du colon; suivie du précis de deux autres observations de blessures, avec lésion du tube intestinal, et produites par armes a feu. Recueil de Memories de Médecine, de Chirurgie et de Pharmacie Militaires (Paris) 7 (1820) 256.

17. Crampton, J. Rupture of the stomach, and escape of its contents into the cavity of the abdomen. London Medical and Physical Journal 39 (1818) 154.

18. Chevalier, T. Case of laceration of the internal coat of the stomach and duodenum, by vomiting. Medico-Chirurgical Transactions 5 (1814) 93.

19. Baillie, D.R. and Travers, B. Review of reference number 17, by Crampton, J. Medico-Chirurgical Transactions 8 (1817) 228.

20. Dupuy, M. Recherches sur la rupture de l'estomac du cheval. Journal de Physiologie Experimentale 1 (1821) 333.

21. Editor. Ulcer in the stomach. Medico-Chirurgical Review 2 (1821–22) 446.

22. Palmer, S. Observations on the diagnosis between central stricture of the stomach, and some of the abdominal lesions with which it may be confounded. The Medico-Chirurgical Journal and Review 1 (1816) 281.

23. Pfeiffer, C.J. (Editor) *Gastric Cancer: Etiology and Pathogenesis*, G. Witzstrock, Baden-Baden and New York, 1979.

24. Editor. Review on practical observations on scirrhus of the stomach, by Bayle and Cayol. Medico-Chirurgical Review 1 (1818–19) 225.

25. Editor. *The Surgeon's Vade Mecum*, Albany, 1813.

26. Brigham, W. Case of long-continued pyloric ulceration, with the appearances on dissection. Medico-Chirurgical Journal 2 (1819–20) 445.

27. Chardel, Dr. General remarks on the treatment of scirrhous affections of the stomach. Medico-Chirurgical Journal 4 (1817) 514.

28. Editor. Remarks by Dr. Abercrombie on scirrhous pylorus. Medico-Chirurgical Review 1 (1824) 191.

29. Editor. M. Broussais' case of cancer of the stomach. The Journal of Foreign Medical Science and Literature 4 (1824) 378.

30. Cheyne, J. Cases of a fetal erethism of the stomach, with observations. The Dublin Hospital Reports and Commentary in Medicine and Surgery 4 (1827) 252.

31. Andral, J. Observations upon excessive dilatation of the stomach, without any obstruction at the pylorus. Collected at the Hospital de la Charité. The Journal of Foreign Medical Science and Literature 3 (1823) 358.

32. Elliotson, J. Cases illustrative of the efficacy of the hydrocyanic or prussic acid in affections of the stomach, with a report upon its powers in pectoral and other diseases in which it has been already recommended, and some facts respecting the necessity of varying the doses of medicines according to circumstances, and the use of opium in diabetes. One Volume, 1820, Reviewed in The Journal of Foreign Medical Science and Literature 1 (1821) 382.

33. Yeats, G.D. An account of the good effects of the white oxide of bismuth in a very severe stomach affection of a gentleman far advanced in years. The Quarterly Journal of Science, Literature, and the Arts 8 (1820) 295.

34. Manley, J.R. Case of irritability of the stomach, attended with alarming symptoms of debility, successfully treated by the internal administration of ice. Medical Repository 6 (1821) 76.

35. Berlioz, Dr. Good effects of evacuations (sanguineous) and acupuncture in chronic diseases. London Medical and Physical Journal 38 (1817) 436.

36. Stone, A.D. *A practical treatise on the diseases of the stomach, and of digestion; including the history and treatment of those affections of the liver and digestive organs, which occur in persons who return from the East and West Indies; with observations on various medicines, and particularly on the improper use of emetics.* 8 vol. pp. 300, London 1806, Reviewed in Medical and Physical Journal 15 (1806) 576.

37. Dewees, W.P. A compendious system of midwifery, chiefly designed to facilitate the inquiries of those who may be pursuing this branch of study, illustrated by occasional cases; with thirteen engravings. 1 vol. pp. 608, Philadelphia, H.C. Carey and I. Lea. Reviewed in The Philadelphia Journal of the Medical and Physical Sciences 9 (1824) 168.

38. Editor. Acids in acidity of the stomach; comment from Dewees' *Midwifery* London Medical and Physical Journal 53 (1825) 350.

39. Dale, J.P. Effects of diet in stomach disorders. Medico-Chirurgical Journal 4 (1817) 40.

40. Baillie, M. *The Morbid Anatomy in Some of the Most Important Parts of the Human Body.* 4th Corrected Edition, W. Bulmer, London, 1812, 470 pp.

41. Powell, R. On certain painful affections of the intestinal canal. The Journal of Foreign Medical Science and Literature 1 (1821) 406.

42. Powell, R. Observations on the bile and its diseases, and on the oeconomy of the liver; read at the Royal College of Physicians, as the Gulstonian Lecture of the Year 1799. The Medical and Chirurgical Review 8 (1801) 242.

43. Ayre, J. *Practical Observations on the Nature and Treatment of Marasmus, and of those Disorders allied to it, which may be strictly denominated Bilious.* London, 1818, 250 pp. Reviewed in Medico-Chirurgical Review 1 (1818-19) 399.

44. Saunders, W. *A Treatise on the Structure, Economy, and Diseases of the Liver; together with an Inquiry into the Properties and Component Parts of the Bile and Biliary Concretions.* 3rd Edition W. Phillips, pp. 342, London 1803.

45. Howship, J. Practical observations on the symptoms, discrimination, and treatment, of some of the most common diseases of the lower intestines, and anus ... London, 176 pages, 1820. Reviewed in The Medico-Chirurgical Review 1 (1820) 222.

46. Calvert, G. A practical treatise on haemorrhoids or piles, strictures and other important diseases of the rectum and anus. The Medico-Chirurgical Review 2 (1825) 273.

47. Yeats, G.D. Some observations on the duodenum, with plates, descriptive of its situation and connexions. The Medico-Chirurgical Review 1 (1820) 639.

48. Editor. Intestinal affections. Medico-Chirurgical Journal 5 (1818) 68.

49. Editor. Review on Researches on the Pathology of the Intestinal Canal by John Abercrombie. Medico-Chirurgical Journal 2 (1819-20) 613.

50. Bougon, M. Observations on a strangulation of the small intestine terminated by gangrene and death. The London Medical and Physical Journal 38 (1817) 169.

51. Brenan, J. Two cases of abdominal obstruction and tendency to inflammation cured by spirits of turpentine, under the management of James Green. London Medical and Physical Journal 36 (1816) 359.

52. Duplan, Dr. Observation d'une hernie estrangler avec gangrene de l'intestin, et querie sans anus artificial. Journal Universel des Sciences Medicales 12 (1818) 101.

53. William, Dr. Miscellaneous works. Medico-Chirurgical Review 3 (1822-23) 51.

54. Monfalcon, M. Case of gastrotomy, with remarks. Medico-Chirurgical Review 1 (1818-19) 255.

55. Editor. Dr. Kennedy's account of morbid concretion. Medico-Chirurgical Journal 4 (1817) 186.

56. Kopfli, Dr. Lacerated ileum, without external marks of violation. Medico-Chirurgical Journal 4 (1817) 137.

57. Andral, J. Researches on the pathological anatomy of the digestive canal. Medico-Chirurgical Review 4 (1823-24) 673.

58. Askwith, W. A case of extensive ulceration of the rectum and colon. London Medical Review 6 (1801) 346.

59. Lettsom, J.C. Case of the vermis lumbricus perforating the intestinal canal and abdomen. The London Medical and Physical Journal 38 (1817) 130.

60. Robertson, A. Case of enteritis, terminating in serous effusion into the abdomen; with the appearances on dissection. Medico-Chirurgical Review 1 (1818–19) 150.

61. Hayes, W. On the cure of chronic diarrhoea, etc. The Philadelphia Medical Museum 1 (1805) 427.

62. Stimson, J. Case of chronic diarrhoea, accompanied by the discharge of some peculiar substances. London Medical and Physical Journal 38 (1817) 193.

63. Editor. Observation on the employment of cupping glasses in obstinate diarrhoea. The Medico-Chirurgical Journal and Review 4 (1817) 337.

64. Ferguson, W. On the mercurial plan of treatment of dysentery. Medico-Chirurgical Transactions 2 (1817) 181.

65. Smith, N.R. *A physiological essay on digestion.* E. Bliss and E. White, New York, pp. 93, 1825. Reviewed in the New York Monthly Chronicle of Medicine and Surgery 1 (1825) 326.

66. Editor. On the different appearances presented by the mucous membrane of the stomach and intestinal canal when in a healthy state. Lancet 1 (1825) 56.

67. Philip, A.P.W. A treatise on indigestion and its consequences, called nervous and bilious complaints, with observations on the organic diseases in which they sometimes terminate. 2nd Edition, London 1822, pp. 391. Reviewed in The Journal of Foreign Medical Science and Literature 2 (1822) 467.

68. Cuvier, de M. Du canal alimentaire et de ses annexes dans les animaux sans vertebres. Bibliothèque Médicale 26 (1807) 149.

69. Home, Mr. Observations, on the structure of the different cavities which constitute the stomach of the whale, compared with those of ruminating animals, with a view to ascertain the situation of the digestive organ. The Philadelphia Medical Museum 4 (1808) 184.

70. Monro, A. Engravings of the thoracic and abdominal viscera, and the canals connected with them; representing the natural appearance of those important parts immediately after death, and without being affected by previous disease. Edinburgh, 1814, pp. 31. The London Medical Repository Monthly Journal and Review 3 (1815) 401.

71. Houlton, J. A treatise on the anatomy and physiology of the mucous membranes; with illustrative pathological observations. London Medical Repository Monthly Journal and Review 16 (1821) 462.

72. Broughton, S.D. Experiments and remarks, illustrating the influence of the eighth pair of nerves over the organs of respiration and digestion. The Quarterly Journal of Science, Literature, and the Arts 10 (1821) 292.

73. Cooper, Sir A. and Philip, W. The process of digestion explained, with experiments on beef, mutton, pork, etc. The Family Oracle of Health, Economy, Medicine and Good Living 1 (1824) 131.

74. Glover, J. An attempt to prove that digestion, in man, depends on the united causes of solution and fermentation. Dissertation, Way and Groff, Philadelphia, pp. 39, 1800.

75. James, J. An essay on indigestion. The Philadelphia Journal of the Medical and Physical Sciences 9 (1824) 1.

76. Montègre, A.J. Sur la digestion dans l'homme. Journal de Médecine, Chirurgie, Pharmacie 31 (1814) 305.

77. Leuret, M. and Lassaigne, M. Recherches physiologiques et chimiques pour servir à l'histoire de la digestion. Revue Médicale (Historique et Philosophique) Paris 20 (1825) 359.

78. Editor. Communication between the stomach and bladder. The Journal of Foreign Medical Science and Literature 3 (1823) 546.

79. Home, E. Experiments of prove that fluids pass directly from the stomach to the circulation of the blood, and thence into the cells of the spleen, the gall bladder, and urinary bladder, without going through the thoracic duct. New York Medical and Philsophical Journal and Review 3 (1811) 244.

80. Kasich, A.M. William Prout and the discovery of hydrochloric acid in the gastric juice. Bulletin of the History of Medicine 20 (1946) 340.

81. Kisch, B. Jacob Anton Helm and William Beaumont. Journal of the History of Medicine and Allied Sciences 22 (1967) 54.

82. Harrison, E. An account of experiments performed with a view to ascertain the effect of the nitric acid upon iron deposited in the stomach of an animal. The Medical and Chirurgical Review 6 (1799-1800) 403.

83. Editor. Extraordinary powers of the human stomach, exemplified in the case of a man who swallowed knives. Medical Repository 1 (1809) 84.

84. Young, J.R. An experimental inquiry into the principles of nutrition and the digestive process (thesis, Univ. of Penn.), Philadelphia, Eaker and Mecum, 1803, pp. 40.

85. Prout, W. On the nature of the acid and saline matters usually existing in the stomachs of animals. Royal Society of London, Philosophical Transactions 144 (1824) 204.

86. Burns, A. Observations on the digestion of the stomach after death. The Eclectic Repertory and Analytical Review, Medical and Philosophical 1 (1811) 193.

87. Editor. Of animal fluids. Medico-Chirurgical Transactions 4 (1813) 77.

88. Graves, R.J. Acid in the human stomach. The Medico-Chirurgical Review 2 (1825) 145.

89. Perperes, M. The nature of acid formed in indigestion. Medical and Physical Journal 20 (1808) 193.

90. Adams, J. *Observations on morbid poisons, chronic and acute.* Callow, London, pp. 405, 1806. Reviewed in The Medico and Chirurgical Review 14 (1807) 25.

91. Beaumont, W. *Experiment and observations on the gastric juice and the physiology of digestion.* Plattsburg, 1833.

92. Fulton, J.F. and Wilson, L.G. *Selected readings in the history of physiology.* Chapter 5, Digestion, 2nd Ed., Charles C. Thomas, Springfield, 1966, pp. 159-200.

93. Helm, J. *Zwey Kranken-Geschichten*, Wien, 1803, and Medical and Physical Journal 11 (1804) 44.

94. Editor. Remarks on the functions of the stomach, and on the singular case related by Jacob Helm, Physician in Vienna, etc., in a letter from Professor Waterhouse to Professor Mitchill, dated Cambridge, March 5, 1808. Medical Repository 6 (1808) 1.

95. Editor. Fistulous wound of the stomach. Medico-Chirurgical Review 1 (1818-19) 264.

96. Scudamore, Dr. Experiments on digestion. Lancet 1 (1824) 134.

97. Lallemand, F. Pathological observations, illustrative of some points in physiology. London Medical and Physical Journal 40 (1818) 531.

98. Marcet, A. Some experiments on the chemical nature of chyle, with a few observations upon chyme. The Medico-Chirurgical Transactions 6 (1819) 618.

99. Andral, J. Researches on the pathological anatomy of the digestive canal, considered in its sub-diaphragmatic portion. The Journal of Foreign Medical Science and Literature 3 (1823) 395.

100. Editor. Observations on the gastric glands of the human stomach, and the contraction which takes place in that viscus. London Medical and Physical Journal 39 (1818) 402.

101. Rush, B. An inquiry into the functions of the spleen, liver, pancreas, and thyroid gland. The Medical and Chirurgical Review 15 (1807) 95.

102. Brodie, B.C. Observations on the effects produced by the bile, in the process of digestion. The Quarterly Journal of Science, Literature and the Arts 14 (1823) 341.

103. Chevruel, M. Sur la presence de la cholesterine dans la bile de l'homme. Journal de Physiologie et Pathologique 4 (1824) 257.

104. Smith, E. *Observations and experiments on the digestive powers of the bile in animals.* Longman and Co., London, 77, 1805. Reviewed in The Medical and Chirurgical Review 13 (1806) 129.

105. Hahn, B. *Observations and experiments on the use of enemata and the external application of medicines to the human body.* Philadelphia, 1798.

106. Hodge, B. Experiments and observations on the absorption of active medicines into the circulation. Philadelphia, 1801.

107. Magendie, F. Mémoire sur le mécanisme de l'absorption chez les animaux a sang rouge et chaud. Journal de Physiologie Experimentale 1 (1821) 1, 18.

108. Editor. Of the present state of our knowledge respecting the function of absorption. The London Medical Repository Monthly Journal and Review. New Series 3 (1825) 1.

109. Bernard, M.C. Mémoire sur le pancrées et sur le role du suc pancréatique dans les phénomènes digestifs, particulièrement dans la digestion des matières grasses neutres. Compt. Rend. Acad. Sci., Suppl. 1 (1856) 379.

Chapter IX

1. Hansen, J.B. and S.A. Pedersen. The relation between barometric pressure and the incidence of perforated duodenal ulcer. Proc. 4th World Congress Gastroenterology, Copenhagen, 1970, p. 97.

2. Editorial, Medical and Physical Journal 27 (1812) 264.

3. Clark J. Medical Notes on Climate, Diseases, Hospitals, and Medical Schools in France, Italy, and Switzerland; comprising an Inquiry into the Effects of a Residence in the South of Europe, in Cases of Pulmonary Consumption, and illustrating the present State of Medicine in those Countries. London, 1820, 250 pp., Reviewed in Medico-Chirurgical Journal 2 (1819-20) 577.

4. Wood, J. Letter to Editor on Seasons attending Epidemics. Medical and Physical Journal 19 (1808) 161.

5. Buxton, T. An Essay on the Use of Regulated Temperature in Winter-Cough and Consumptions; including a Comparison of the different Methods of producing such a Temperature in the Chambers of Invalids. Medical and Physical Journal 23 (1810) 150.

6. Speer. On the Diseases of the Lower Orders in Dublin. The Dublin Hospital Reports and Communications in Medicine and Surgery 3 (1822) 170.

7. Robertson, J. Report on the Diseases of Edinburgh for January, 1809. Medical and Physical Journal 21 (1809) 258.

8. Lind. J. An Essay on Diseases incidental to Europeans in Hot Climates, with the Method of preventing their fatal Consequence. Sixth Edition, Richardson, London, 1809, Reviewed in Medical and Physical Journal 21 (1809) 71.

9. Pearson, A. Some Observations on the Pathology and Prevailing Diseases of Hot Climates. Medical and Physical Journal 13 (1805) 481.

10. Pearson, A. Some Observations on the Pathology and Prevailing Diseases of Hot Climates. Medical and Physical Journal 11 (1804) 200.

11. Alder, T. Letter to Editor. Medical and Physical Journal 15 (1806) 40.

12. Alder, T. Proofs of the Proximate and Remote Causes of Diseases and Fevers. Medical and Physical Journal 23: 116, 281, and 469:1810.

13. Editorial. Project for relieving Disorders of the Human Constitution by diminishing the Pressure of the Atmosphere upon it. Medical Repository 5 (1802) 473.

14. Folwell, Observations on the Influence of the Moon on Climate and the Animal Economy; with a proper Method of treating Diseases with under the Power of that Luminary. Philadelphia, 24 pp., 1798, Reviewed in Medical Repository 4 (1801) 285.

15. Balfour. Treatise on Sol-Lunar Influence in Fevers. 2nd Edition, London, 1795.

16. Bell, J. On Periodicity and Lunar Influence in Diseases. The Philadelphia Journal of the Medical and Physical Sciences 11 (1825) 61.

17. Tranziere, D.A. Memoir on a periodical Difficulty of Breathing, tending to prove the Influence of the Moon on the human Body. Medical and Physical Journal 8 (1802) 401.

18. Colhoun, S. On the Medical Character of the United States. The Philadelphia Journal of the Medical and Physical Sciences 2 (1821) 39.

19. Bradstreet. On the Proximate Cause of Fever. Medical Commonwealth of the Massachusetts Medical Society 3 (1822) 290.

20. Editor. Atmospheric Constitution and Diseases of New York. Medical Repository 4 (1818) 421.

21. Wilson, J. An Inquiry into the Nature and Treatment of the prevailing Epidemic, called Spotted Fever. Bradford and Read, Boston, 216 pp., 1815. Reviewed in Medical Repository 3 (1817) 253.

Chapter X

1. Jackson, R. *An Exposition of the Practice of Affusing Cold Water on the Surface of the Body, as a Remedy for the Cure of Fever; to which are added, Remarks on the Effects of Cold Drink, and of Gestation in the open Air, in certain Conditions of that Disease.* Edinburgh, 1808. Reviewed in Medical and Physical Journal 20 (1808) 81.

2. Editor. On the employment of cold externally (Taken from Journal de Med. et des Sc. Access) Lancet 4 (1824) 400.

3. Buchan, W. *Domestic Medicine, or A Treatise on the Prevention and Cure of Diseases, by Regimen and Simple Medicines: with Observations on Sea-Bathing, and the Use of the Mineral Waters.* London, 1826, 22 Edition.

4. Macenzie, P. *Practical Observations on the Medicinal Powers of Mineral Waters, and of the various Modes of Bathing, etc., with Remarks on Exercise and Diet.* Medico-Chirurgical Review 1 (1820) 605.

5. Coffin, J.G. *Discourses on Cold and Warm Bathing with Remarks on the Effects of Drinking Cold Water in Warm Weather.* Boston, 1818. Reviewed in Medical Repository 6 (1821) 450.

6. Howship, J. Observations and cases illustrative of the effects produced by the solar heat upon the human body. Medical and Physical Journal 23 (1810) 193.

7. Editor. Diseases of August, and the means of escaping them. The Family Oracle of Health, Economy, Medicine, and Good Living 2 (1825) 7.

8. Welsh, T. A dissertation read before the Massachusetts Medical Society on heat and cold. Medical Commentary of the Massachusetts Medical Society 2 (1813) 286.

9. Chapman, N. Thoughts on animal heat. Philadelphia Journal of the Medical and Physical Sciences 7 (1823) 23.

10. Henry, W. A review of some experiments which have been supposed to disprove the materiality of heat. The Philosophical Magazine 15 (1803) 45.

11. Tupper, M. Observations on animal heat. Medical and Physical Journal 8 (1802) 500.

12. Earle, H. Cases and observations, illustrating the influence of the nervous system in regulating animal heat. Medico-Chirurgical Transactions 7 (1816) 173.

13. Davy, J. An account of some experiments on animal heat. The Eclectic Repertory and Analytical Review of Medicine and Philosophy 6 (1816) 183.

14. Davy, J. On the heat evolved during the coagulation of blood. The London Medical Repository, Monthly Journal, and Review 7 (1817) 320.

15. Pearson, A. Some observations on the pathology and prevailing diseases of warm climates. Medical and Physical Journal 11 (1804) 158.

16. Anonymous. Letter to editors, on cold water in gout. Medical and Physical Journal 11 (1804) 150.

17. Taylor, T. Letter to editors, on cold water in gout. Medical and Physical Journal 11 (1804) 346.

18. Anonymous. Letter to editors, on cold affusion in gout. Medical and Physical Journal 11 (1804) 521.

19. Anonymous. Letter to editors, on cold bathing in rheumatism. Medical and Physical Journal 9 (1803) 549.

20. Pfeiffer, C.J., Cho, C.H., Cheema, A., and Saltman, D. Reserpine-induced gastric ulcers: protection by lysomal stabilization due to zinc. European Journal of Pharmacology 61 (1980) 347.

21. Pfeiffer, C.J., Cho, C.H. Modulating effect by zinc on hepatic lysosomal fragility induced by surface-active agents. Research Communications in Chemical Pathology and Pharmacology 27 (1980) 587.

22. Johnson, P. On the good effects of cold applications to ulcers. The New England Journal of Medicine and Surgery 4 (1815) 156.

23. M'Dowell, Dr. Cold, as a remedy for scalds, Medical Repository 2 (1810) 286.

24. Kinglake, Dr. Cases of the cooling treatment of burns and scalds, Medical and Physical Journal 16 (1806) 17, 460, and 526.

25. Dzondi, Dr. On burns, London Medical and Physical Journal 36 (1816) 245.

26. Little D. Letter to editors, on strangulated hernia. Medical and Physical Journal 17 (1807) 55.

27. Wray, S. Cases illustrating the decided efficacy of cold affusion in the treatment of poisoning from opium, The New England Journal of Medicine and Surgery 12 (1823) 92.

28. Heim, Prof. On the applying of cold water in the cure of hydrocephalus, The London Medical Repository, Monthly Journal, and Review 5 (1816) 75.

29. Brown, G.G. The efficacy of cold in madness. Medical Repository 4 (1801) 209.

30. Lodge, T. Remarks on the efficacy of cold affusion in typhus and scarlet fever, London Medical and Physical Journal 33 (1815) 358.

31. Anonymous. Letter to the editors, on typhus, Medical and Physical Journal 16 (1807) 236.

32. Wright, W. On the external use of cold water in the small-pox, Medical and Physical Journal 19 (1808) 272.

33. Ryal, J. Letter to the editors, on cold affusion in colic, Medical and Physical Journal 8 (1805) 18.

34. Thackeray, W.M. Letter to the editors, on cold water in convulsions, Medical and Physical Journal 7 (1804) 508.

35. Currey, G.G. A case of tetanus arising from a wound, in which the affusion of cold water was successfully employed, Medical Transactions 4 (1813) 166.

36. Harris, W. A case of tetanus cured by the cold bath, Medical Repository 4 (1801) 76.

37. Dewar, H. Letter to the editors, on cold ablution. Medical and Physical Journal 11 (1804) 21.

38. Utley, V. A dissertation on the cold practice, in febrile diseases, Medical Repository 5 (1820) 36.

39. Shillito, C. On the effects of immersion in the sea in intermittent fever, The London Medical Repository, Monthly Journal, and Review 9 (1818) 364.

40. Editor. Philosophy of bathing, cold bath and affusion in fevers, The Family Oracle of Health, Economy, Medicine, and Good Living 2 (1825) 381.

41. Anonymous. On the efficacy of the cold affusion in cutting short the paroxysm of certain convulsive diseases. Medico-Chirurgical Journal 4 (1817) 249.

42. Nicholl, A. Experiments and observations on the tepid, warm, and hot baths, The London Medical Repository, Monthly Journal, and Review 9 (1818) 130.

43. Editor. Some historical account of the progress of medical science, The New England Journal of Medicine and Surgery 3 (1814) 5.

44. Editor. Hot water a remedy for hysteria. Medical Repository 7 (1822) 112.

45. Marsh, H. A brief notice of the effects of the vapour bath in tetanus. The Dublin Hospital Reports and Commentary in Medicine and Surgery 4 (1827) 567.

46. Jennings, S. A plain elementary explanation of the nature and cure of diseases, predicated upon facts and experience; presenting a view of that train of thinking which led to the invention of the patent portable warm and hot bath. Richmond, 1814. Reviewed in Medical Repository 2 (1815) 368.

47. Teallier, N. Case showing the effects of a very hot and prolonged bath, in a case of chronic rheumatism. The London Medical Repository, Monthly Journal, and Review 3 (1825) 164.

48. Dexter, A. Dissertation on the use of blisters in diseases of the articulations. Medical Commentary of the Massachusetts Medical Society 2 (1813) 301.

49. Killett, M. Observations on the use of nitrous acid as a substitute for blisters. The Journal of Foreign Medical Science and Literature 1 (1821) 492.

50. Kinglake, Dr. On blistering and topical cold, London Medical and Physical Journal 38 (1817) 102.

51. Syer, J. Remarks on the administration of blisters, The London Medical Repository, Monthly Journal, and Review 7 (1817) 105.

52. Smith, J.A. A case of mortification arrested by the application of blisters, New York Medical and Philosophical Journal and Review 1 (1809) 175.

53. Baillie, M. The case of a boy seven years of age, who had hydrocephalus, in whom

some of the bones of the skull once firmly united, were, in the progress of the disease, separated to a considerable distance from each other. Medical Transactions 4 (1813) 1.

54. Blane, Sir G. Remarks on the preceding case of cynanche laryngea, Medico-Chirurgical Transactions 6 (1815) 141.

55. Anonymous. Ileus, Medico-Chirurgical Review 1 (1818-1819) 131.

56. Pearson, A. Some observations on the pathology and prevailing diseases of warm climates, Medical and Physical Journal 11 (1804) 200.

Chapter XI

1. Howard-Jones, N. Man and his medicines, *World Health*, April 4-11 (1974).

2. Chapman, N. *Elements of Therapeutics and Materia Medica*, Vols. 1 & 2, Fifth Edition, Philadelphia, Carey, Lea, and Carey, 1827, pp. 52-87, (Vol. 1).

3. Urdang, G. Pharmacopoeias as witnesses of world history, J. Hist. Med. 1 (1946) 46-69.

4. Corlett, W.T. *The Medicine Man of the American Indian*, New York, 1935, p. 318.

5. Sonnedecker, G. (Reviser), Kremera and Urdang's *History of Pharmacy*, 4th Ed., J.B. Lippincott Co., Phil., 1976, pp. 1-571.

6. Berman, A. The scientific tradition in French hospital pharmacy. Am. J. Hosp. Pharm. 18 (1961) 110.

7. Wesley, A.M. *Primitive Physic: or, An Easy and Natural Method of Curing Most Diseases*, 26th Edition, Geo. Story, London, 1807.

8. Alexander, D. Dissertation on the means of preserving health. Medico-Chirurgical Transactions, 2, 2-14 (1800).

9. Reece, R. *The Medical Guide, for the Use of the Clergy, Heads of Families, and Junior Practitioners in Medicine and Surgery*. 14th Edition, Longman, Hurst, Rees, Orme, Brown and Green, London, 1824, pp. 1-414.

10. Sweetser, W.S. On the treatment of cynanche trachealis; being part of a dissertation on that disease, which obtained the Boylston Prize for 1820. The New-England Journal of Medicine and Surgery 10 (1821) 1-16.

11. Jeffreys, H. Cases in surgery, selected from the records of the author's practice at the St. George's and St. James Dispensary; and illustrating the nature and mode of treatment of strumous or scrofulous ophthalmia; the sedative powers of tartar emetic in the cure of local inflammations, when administered internally; the treatment of the mammary, or milk abscess; and the beneficial effects of elm bark as a cheap substitute for sarsaparilla. Reviewed in Medico-Chirurgical Review 3 (1822-23) 535-545.

12. Hallar, J.S., Jr. The use and abuse of tartar emetic in the 19th-century materia medica. Bull. Hist. Med. 49 (1975) 235-257.

13. Alder, Dr. Proofs of the proximate causes of diseases from the practice of physic. Medical and Physical Journal 22 (1809) 458-464.

14. Balfour, William. *Observations, with cases, illustrative of the sedative and febrifuge powers of emetic tartar*. Octavo, one volume, 92 pp. London, 1818, Reviewed in Medico-Chirurgical Review 1 (1818-19) 358-360.

15. Smith, J.M. Efficacy of emetics in spasmodic diseases. Medico-Chirurgical Review 2 (1821-22) 282-314.

16. Tynicola, Dr. Letter to editor, Dr. Bradley, Medical and Physical Journal 8 (1802) 64-77.

17. Winterbottom, R. Letter to editor, Dr. Bradley, Medical and Physical Journal 11 (1804) 78-81.

18. Rees, George. *A Practical Treatise on Haemoptysis, or Spitting of Blood: Shewing the Safety and Efficacy of Emetics, and the Pernicious Effect of Blood-letting, in the Treatment of that Disease*, London, 48 pp. Reviewed in The New England Journal of Medicine and Surgery 5 (1816) 99-102.

19. Hosack, Dr. Emetics in constipation, Medico-Chirurgical Review 3 (1822-23) 410-412.

20. Lyon, E. Practical observations on certain inflammatory affections of the mucous membranes of the lungs and alimentary canal. Medico-Chirurgical Review 1 (1824) 172–175.

21. Sharkey, Dr. On the use of emetics in pulmonary consumption, Medical and Physical Journal 19 (1808) 337–344.

22. Moerker, Dr. A case report on use of emetic tartar for removal of a piece of beef stuck in the fauces. Medical and Physical Journal 11 (1804) 190–192.

23. Chapman, Dr. On emetics, as counteracting salivation, The Journal of Foreign Medical Science and Literature 4 (1824) 210–211.

24. Beyerle, Dr. Induration and contraction of the stomach. Medico-Chirurgical Journal 4 (1817) 332–334.

25. Barton, B. Letter to Dr. Ramsay, in consequence of his observations on the bite of a snake cured by volatile alkali, Medical and Physical Journal 11 (1804) 334–337.

26. Balfour, W. Observations on the internal use of nitrate of silver, Medico-Chirurgical Journal 5 (1818) 464–470.

27. Badeley, Dr. On the effect of nitrate of silver on the complexion. (Communicated by Sir H. Halford). Medico-Chirurgical Transactions 9 (1818) 234–239.

28. Editor. Physiology, surgery, and practice of medicine, The London Medical Repository, Monthly Journal and Review 3 (1815) 144–145.

29. Armstrong, Dr. Chronic diseases, Medico-Chirurgical Review, N.S., 1 (1818–19) 55–62.

30. Robertson, H. Of the effect of mercury on the living body, The London Medical Repository, Monthly Journal and Review, N.S., 1 (1824) 457–464.

31. Pfeiffer, C.J. Gastroenterologic response to environmental agents—absorption and interactions (Chapt. 22, pp. 355–357) and Pfeiffer, C.J. and Hänninen, O. Alimentary excretion of environmental agents and unnatural compounds (Chapt. 33, pp. 524–525), in Lee, D.H.K. (Editor) *Reactions to Environmental Agents, Handbook of Physiology*, American Physiological Society, 1977, Bethesda.

32. Paris, J.A. *Pharmacologia; or, the History of Medicinal Substances, with a View to Establish the Art of Prescribing and of Composing Extemporaneous Formulae upon Fixed and Scientific Principles: Illustrated by Formulae, in which the Intention of Each Element is Designated by Key Letters.* 3rd Ed., London, 432 pp., Reviewed in Medico-Chirurgical Review 1 (1820) 80–97.

33. Hermant, M. Sur une méthode simple, facile et prompte de guéris les affections syphilitiques, *Recueil de Memories de Medecine, de Chirurgie et de Pharmacie Militaires (Paris)* 6 (1819) 320–329.

34. Davies, D. An essay on mercury; wherein are presented formulae for some preparations of this metal, including practical remarks on the safest and most effectual methods of administering them, for the cure of liver complaints, dropsies, syphilis, and other formidable diseases incident to the human frame; being the result of long experience and diligent observation. London, 1820, 35 pp., Reviewed in Medico-Chirurgical Review 1 (1820) 700–702.

35. Hamilton, J. *Observations on the Use and Abuse of Mercurial Medicines in Various Diseases*, Edinburgh, 1819, 222 pp.

36. Thomson, H. *An Inquiry into the Effects of Mercury on the Human Body, with a View to Estimate its Value as a Remedy in Several Important Diseases*, London, 1820, 56 pp.

37. Bacot, J. *Observations on Syphilis, principally with Reference to the Use of Mercury in that Disease*, London, 1821, 115 pp.

38. Francis, J.W. Dissertation on quicksilver medically considered. Medical Repository 1 (1813) 71–76.

39. Wheaton, L. Some further remarks on the use of mercury in fevers. Medical Repository 1 (1809) 139–144.

40. Boyle, J. Observations on large doses of submuriate of mercury for the cure of syphilis. Medico-Chirurgical Journal 5 (1818) 197–201.

41. Porter, W.H. Case of cynanche laryngea in which tracheotomy and mercury were successfully employed: with remarks. Medico-Chirurgical Transactions 11 (1821) 414–439.

42. Carmichael, R. *An Essay on the Venereal Diseases which have been confounded with*

Syphilis, and the Symptoms which exlusively arise from that Poison. Gilbert and Hodges, Dublin, 1814, 121 pp., Reviewed in The London Medical Repository, Monthly Journal and Review 4 (1815) 313–324.

43. Moseley, Dr. On the prevention and cure of canine madness. Medical Repository 6 (1808) 383–385.

44. Bardsley, Dr. Experiments with the white oxide of bismuth. The Philadelphia Medical and Philosophical Register 4 (1807) 162–171.

45. Anonymous. Case of chronic hydrocephalus, Medico-Chirurgical Journal 4 (1817) 81–82.

46. Anonymous. Case of tumors of the tongue cured by mercury. Medical and Physical Journal 26 (1811) 494–495.

47. Editor. Excerpt on mercury from The Edinburgh Journal, Medical and Physical Journal 28 (1810) 520–521.

48. Black, E. Letter to Editor, S.L. Mitchell, dated Nov. 1, 1808, on Consumption of the Lungs. Medical Repository 1 (1809) 116–125.

49. Chisholme, C. Two examples of the beneficial effects of mercury in some severe affections of the brain. Medico-Chirurgical Transactions 4 (1813) 35–37.

50. Wright, Dr. Mercury in acute diseases, Medico-Chirurgical Review 4 (1823–24) 222.

51. Armstrong, Dr. Efficacy of mercury in congestive typhus. Medico-Chirurgical Journal 3 (1817) 175.

52. Mease, J. Case of the successful use of mercury in typhus; with observations on its use in tetanus. Medical and Physical Journal 19 (1808) 109–112.

53. Sheppard, J.B. On the mercurial treatment of yellow fever. The New England Journal of Medicine and Surgery 7 (1818) 247–258.

54. Davies, D.H. Letter to the Editor, Medical and Physical Journal 26 (1811) 277–278.

55. Miccoli, Dr. Stibiated mercurial ointment, Medico-Chirurgical Review 1 (1824) 230–234.

56. Astbury, J. Cases of the effects of mercury on the heart, The New-England Journal of Medicine and Surgery, 8 (1819) 173–175.

57. Stringham, J.S. On the diuretic effects of mercury in a case of syphilis. Medical and Physical Journal 18 (1807) 331–340.

58. Guthrie, G.J. Remarks on certain opinions and doctrines relative to the phagedenic ulcer contained in Mr. Carmichael's late work on venereal disease. Medico-Chirurgical Review 1 (1818–19) 323–340.

59. Editor. Analytical review on syphilis, pseudo-syphilis, and mercury. Medico-Chirurgical Review 2 (1821–22) 597–626.

Index

233